Dystonia:
The Disease that Distorts

EUGENE SMITH

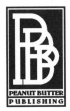

PEANUT BUTTER
PUBLISHING

Seattle, Washington
Portland, Oregon
Denver, Colorado
Vancouver, B.C.

ISBN # 0-89716-621-3
LOC 96-68617
11.0056
Cover design: David Marty
Production: Elizabeth Lake

First printing April 1996
Second printing April 1998
10 9 8 7 6 5 4 3 2 1

Peanut Butter Publishing
226 2nd Avenue West • Seattle, WA 98119
Old Post Office Bldg. • 510 S.W. 3rd • Portland, OR 97201
Cherry Creek • 50 S. Steele • Suite 850 • Denver, CO 80209
Su. 230 1333 Johnston St. Pier 32 Granville Isl.,Vancouver, B.C.
V6H 3R9
e mail: P NUT PUB@aol.com
http://www.pbpublishing.com
Printed in Canada

To my wife, Marcia,
and to our children,
Sheila, Kenna, Maynard, Bradley, and Naomi,
with gratitude

ACKNOWLEDGMENT

The first printing of this book was underwritten by Medtronic Neurological, manufacturer of the baclofen pump used by some dystonia patients. Both Medtronic and Athena Neurosciences--manufacturer of NeuroBloc, another treatment for dystonia to be available in 1999-- made grants to cover costs of the second printing. The author and the Dystonia Medical Research Foundation are most grateful for their generosity. Because of that generosity, all proceeds from sale of the book help to fund research supported by the Foundation.

Preface

Much of the information about dystonia reported in this book comes directly from interviews. I am grateful to more than 35 dystonia patients from the United States and Canada who allowed me to tape record my conversations with them and gave permission for me to use excerpts from those conversations. I have given each a pseudonym in order to spare them any possible discomfort or embarrassment beyond what they already experience from their dystonia symptoms.

I have identified by name and work site the professional people whom I interviewed and who gave permission for quoting their words.

Foreword

In support groups throughout the United States and Canada, and in twenty other countries in Europe, Asia, South America, and Australia, people with dystonia gather to share experiences. By talking about how dystonia has affected their lives, they gain insight, understanding, and courage.

In this book, we have a valuable and much-needed extension of these support-group conversations. Eugene Smith has interviewed dystonia patients from many geographic regions in the United States and Canada, compiling a representative sample of types of dystonia as it affects both young and older people. He has arranged excerpts from their stories to provide a remarkable introduction to dystonia from the patient's point of view.

I believe this is a book that dystonia patients and their families will be interested in and will want to recommend to others.

Dennis Kessler, President
Dystonia Medical Research Foundation

Table of Contents

Chapter 1

Noticing Mysterious Symptoms

You think you have normal control over all your muscles—your arm, your neck, your eyes, your foot, your vocal cords—till one day you notice that one or more of these muscles is misbehaving. It becomes tense when you perform an ordinary act like writing. Or, the muscles that control the blinking of your eyes pull the eyelids shut for varying periods of time. Or the head starts drifting left or right—pulled by muscles in your neck—and stays off-center. You can even feel spasms in the muscles of the neck and upper back—increasingly painful spasms.

What's going on? Did you exercise too vigorously? Did you sleep "wrong"? Did you take some medication that is producing an unexpected side-effect?

These and hundreds of other persistent questions will nag you over the coming days ... weeks ... months ... years. You'll see physicians who will order blood tests, urinalysis, MRIs, X-rays, CT scans and every other test they can think of. The results from all those tests will probably come back "normal." You and your doctor are no closer than you were many days and hundreds, thousands of dollars ago to knowing what's ailing you.

What, indeed, is going on? Maybe it's "in your head," as we're fond of saying when we're bewildered about some hard-to-diagnose physical problem. Maybe some trauma to your psyche when you were a child is only now expressing itself—causing your eyelid to close when you don't want it to or wrenching your neck around at an odd and extremely annoying angle. Or maybe your voice is sounding choked and raspy because of continual "stage fright" or worse, emotional baggage that can find no other outlet. You've become uptight in every sense!

With no accurate diagnosis and no answer to your questions, you feel trapped and uncertain. It's the uncertainty and the accompanying bewilderment that makes the situation especially hard. With all our elaborate and expensive medical technology, why can't someone get a fix on your problem and tell you what to do about it? What should you do next? Try still another doctor? But which specialty? Try alternative medicine—acupuncture, biofeedback, hypnosis, herbs? Physical therapy? Or just put up with the problem, dealing with it day to day the best you can?

It doesn't go away, most likely, though you begin to notice that, when you first wake up after a night's sleep, your muscles seem normal—at least for a few minutes: the tension is gone; the muscle is under your control and does what it's supposed to do. But only for a blessed, short time. As soon as you get out of bed and begin your day's routine activities, that peculiar muscle misbehavior is back—just like yesterday—maybe not quite as severe as it was late yesterday afternoon but definitely noticeable.

And so it goes. Throughout the day, you make little adjustments to favor the tight, misbehaving muscle. Nothing really helps, even if you can get by and manage not to bump into things or trip over yourself or squeak out what you **must** say. You begin to tell yourself that it's always going to be this way—from now on, you'll feel like a freak, a klutz, a person visited by a mysterious disorder that no one has ever heard of or can identify.

A version of this scenario has occurred to thousands of people—children and adults, all age groups, all ethnicities, all socio-economic levels. I'm one of this group. I have dystonia.

But it's not primarily my story—my experience with having dystonia for over 25 years—that I tell in this book. Instead, I have combined portions of the stories of people from the United States and Canada, most of whom I have interviewed, many with far worse cases of dystonia than mine. I have tried to tell a composite story of dystonia: its curious and often debilitating forms and its effects on people's lives. For at least one person, it "ruined my life." For some, having dystonia has caused years-long pain, frustration, and anger. For others, it has brought to the surface unsuspected strengths and resilience. For everyone who has this disease that distorts their muscles, forcing them into spasms, the cause remains a mystery—a mysterious affliction that turns an otherwise normal life into a lifelong contest with muscles that won't behave.

Chapter 2

Looking Closely at Early Symptoms

Symptoms of dystonia can appear at almost any age—from early childhood to late adulthood. For each person, these symptoms are likely to be different: different in the location and way a specific muscle is affected and different in the speed and manner of the symptoms' progression.

Peter was nearly 13 at the time I interviewed him. An intelligent and extremely articulate boy, he lives in upstate New York and attends public schools. To look at him, you would not suspect that there is anything physically wrong with him, but that's because of his current medication. He has two older brothers who also have dystonia, and his father is a physician who knows a great deal about this movement disorder. Peter is therefore extremely unusual to be growing up with dystonia in an environment of knowledge about it.

Tell me about the first symptoms you noticed.

Well, I was in third grade so I was 7 years old and it was during the summer and what I felt was my left leg—my calf muscle—would cramp up to a point where it would hurt and it'd be hard for me to bend my knees.

Cramp up so much it was really painful?

Yes. Well, I mean it would hurt, so I mean I didn't know if I hurt my muscle or something, so when my father told me that I might have dystonia, it frightened me and after that the symptoms kept on going and it turned out that I did have dystonia.

Now you'd seen dystonia in your brothers before that, hadn't you?

Yes.

So you knew what to expect?

Right.

Why did it frighten you, then?

Well, just because I knew how it was affecting my brothers, and I was afraid that, you know, I could be that ... I could be that bad or even worse than how they were. So I was ...

Had your parents prepared you for this beforehand? I mean had they told you that you might get it too?

Uhh, they told me about it but they figured that, since my brother got it at about seven, and I was eight at this point that ... you know, if I was going to find out, it would be very soon. So when I started feeling cramping, I was like uh-oh, and I got frightened.

Describe the cramping a little more, would you?

Well, I ... it almost felt like that someone was just stretching my muscles almost to like where I had no control over it. It just began to happen so that ... I'd rub it, I'd do everything, I'd sleep with a heating pad, and nothing worked. So when my dad figured maybe I had dystonia, he put me on this first medicine, which did nothing. And I had just been taking Tylenol and Advil in the beginning, so that was just ... felt like I had a sprained ankle or something when I was walking, but uh ...

Were you feeling it all the time, or did it come and go?

It came and went away. When I was nervous about anything, it was really bad—like twice as bad. So I figured maybe it was just, you know, something nervous, but I mean, when it happened and I was just feeling fine, then I knew something must be wrong.

What might you be nervous about to bring it on, especially?

Uhh, I don't know, tests.

So it happened in school a lot?

Yeah, I'd be sitting at my desk and maybe I'd, you know, my teacher would be collecting my homework and I may have forgot to have done my homework or something, and it'd start to hurt me. It just ... lots of different things maybe happened.

And you said this was only in one leg— your left leg?

My left leg.

And you weren't getting any symptoms like that at all in the right?

Right.

Did it start moving up your leg?

Yeah, it began to affect my knee and then up to my thighs, then basically it just ... you know, it got worse and worse and worse until I figure when I was walking one day and I noticed my left foot wasn't pointing forward. It was pointing like this [turns his foot to point inwards] as I was walking, and it was really difficult for me to put my leg where I wanted to put it, and that's when we first really assumed that I had dystonia.

Did you start using a cane or a crutch?

Uhh, no, I just walked for a while and then after a year, when all the medicines did nothing, it got so bad that I had to use crutches because otherwise I couldn't walk at all.

———

Peter has a genetic form of dystonia—called *primary dystonia*—which affects several muscles in the body, usually starting in a leg and progressing upwards to the torso, arms, and head. It is also referred to as *generalized dystonia* and *idiopathic torsion dystonia*. (*Idiopathic* means that the cause is unknown; *torsion* refers to the involuntary turning of a body part—arm, leg, neck, torso, etc.—because of muscular tension.)

Julian is in his early 30s. A tall, fit-looking man, he lives near New York City, where he is employed in an office job with a large company. He looks perfectly normal now, again because of a treatment that controls the symptoms but does not affect the underlying malady.

When did you first notice some symptoms of muscles that weren't behaving properly?

It was August of 1985. I was getting headaches—really excessive headaches. I'd just come back from summer vacation.

How old were you then?

I was 23. I was engaged to be married, and all of a sudden I started getting these headaches and then all of a sudden it started into getting a neckache. Over the course of two weeks my head started tilting to the one side—to the right-hand side. It kept on going more and more, and I'm saying, "Maybe I slept wrong or maybe I have some kind of headache-type thing."

Did you have the headache all day long?

The headache in the beginning was all day long. Then it was decreasing more as the neck would go over.

Was the ache in the front part of your head?

I'd say temple headaches. And then, before I knew it, my head was stuck on my right shoulder. I had no idea what was going on. Didn't have a clue.

Pain in the neck?

Good pain in the neck. [laughs] It had to be the worst experience I've ever had in my life. My right shoulder had gone up and my head had gone all the way to the right.

Did you have muscle spasms associated with the pain?

Spasms were like ... uhhh ... how can you explain them? It's almost like when you sleep on your side in a certain way and you wake up and you're ... or if you go to sleep and your leg all of a sudden jumps ... that's exactly what it's like. It happens, you know, 1500 times a day. That's the only difference.

Julian describes the kind of sensation we often call a charley horse, but, unlike the occasional charley horse that anyone might have, the spasms of dystonia seldom go away. His neck or back spasms and his head-turning, resulting from extreme contraction of his dystonic muscles, identify a common type of focal dystonia: *cervical dystonia* (*cervical* refers to the neck), also called *spasmodic torticollis*. *Torticollis* means turning of the head. *Spasmodic* refers to the jerking effect of muscles involuntarily contracting, partially relaxing, and then contracting again.

Anna's dystonia involving her head took a different form from Julian's.

When did you first notice that you had something with your muscles that wasn't quite what you considered normal?

I think it was 1979—sometime in 1979. The first time I noticed it was right at this table, sitting where you're sitting [in the kitchen of the home on Long Island, New York, that she shares with her husband]. I was helping my son with his homework, and he was in high school, I think. And I felt my head going back and forth as if I were saying no. And I remember saying to myself, "It's a lousy habit you're getting into. If you don't want to do it, just don't do it." In other words, I thought I was angry that I was helping him, and perhaps I was. That was the first that I noticed it. No, I'm lying. That was the first time after the first time. The first time was coming out of surgery in '76, I think. I had had three surgical procedures in three months.

And when I was able to sit up, each time I sat up my head would shake back and forth in this "no" way.

There was no pain associated with this?

There was no pain associated with it at all.

Just a lack of control?

Lack of control. Lack of muscle control, and they told me it was surgical fatigue. It would go away in about three days.

Was the surgery in the same area?

No. No, no, no. It was unrelated, totally unrelated.

Apparently, then, from what you've said it was a gentle sort of shake, as though you were saying no. It wasn't a tight-spasm shake. Is that right?

After the surgery, it was more radical. You know, I mean I knew I was shaking. I couldn't keep my head straight, but when it began the second time ... when it began in '79 it was very gentle, and only I knew I was doing it because, when I realized I was doing it all the time, I decided—in my infinite wisdom—that, if nobody saw, it didn't count, and I wasn't going to do anything about it until the following spring when there was an evening at the synagogue in which we were being honored. And a very dear friend—who's known me since I'm about 29—said to my daughter, "Why is your mother shaking? What's the matter with her?" My daughter had a fit and said, "There's nothing the matter with my mother." And about a week or two later, she said to me, "Do you know what she said? 'You're shaking.' There's something the matter?"

I said, "Well, I am." So then I had to pay a little attention to it on a more major scale.

And then from the shaking there was a progression so that there was some pain or a tighter turning of the head?

It was tight and then I started going to the doctor, and he gave me Parafon Forte for a muscle relaxant. And then it let up. It let up, and I wasn't as aware of it and I didn't pay much attention to it. Then the next year it came back. This is the time of year [Spring] it seems to ... but it came back and I know now that I react to the increased intensity of the light—of the natural light. So it came back and then we treated it and then we went on to something else. I went to another doctor, went on Inderal. A neurologist gave me Inderal, and I decided that was not for me, and it kept breaking through. Then it got radical. In the kitchen one day we were talking, and, whatever, it was toward evening. There was darkness and white walls and what-have-you—a lot going on around, but I know now the variable light sets me off and all of a sudden my head just started going back and forth and back and forth.

Anna's complex combination of erratic muscular behavior suggests that her dystonia is also *cervical*, though manifesting differently from Julian's.

Lillian, also in late middle age and a resident of the Greater New York City area, has a form of dystonia that mostly affects the small muscles around her eyes.

Your dystonia is limited to the eye area?

To the eye area basically and sometimes I get some sort of movement in the cheeks.

And for how long have you experienced this?

Sixteen years.

How did it start? What were the feelings when it started?

It started with ptosis—drooping of the upper eyelid—of my left eye. It started to close involuntarily and went on like that for quite a while and then it gradually progressed. It got pretty bad. The blepharospasm [the term for the form of dystonia that affects the muscles that control the eyelids] per se disabled me to the point where I could not function as well as I would like to have functioned. I couldn't read. I couldn't watch television. I still can't till this day. Oddly enough, when I paint—I do some painting—I seem to be quiet. At that point, it seems to quiet down. So I assume that if you like something, you enjoy doing something, that helps. It doesn't last too long. I mean you can't stay with anything too long because the eyes start pulling. I've learned to force them to stay open, which creates a tremendous pain across the forehead—literally force them.

Do you tense the muscles to widen the eyes?

Exactly. Can't keep that up too long. So by the end of each day I'm a total wreck. It's gotten progressively worse. In the beginning, the mornings weren't too bad, and then as the day progressed, the spasms would be worse. I was caught one time trying to cross a street, and I went into a spasm in the middle of the street, so I had to take both fingers and pull to try to release them. Those muscles get very strong. And finally I made it. But it's disorienting, debilitating. It's destructive. It's depressing—especially someone who has been active all my life, such as I have been, and then all of a sudden you're kind of limited in what you can do.

The name for Lillian's form of dystonia—*blepharospasm*—means, literally, spasm of the eyelid. It must be distinguished from two other terms for disorders of the eyelid: *blepharitis*, which means inflammation of the eyelid, and *conjunctivitis*, which means inflammation of the mucous membrane inside the eyelid. Each can cause abnormal behavior of the eyelid, but neither is a type of dystonia.

For Andre, who grew up in Winnepeg, Manitoba, and still lives there, signs of "motor difficulty," as he calls it, started appearing when he was about thirteen years old.

What were your early symptoms?

When writing with any perceived stress, like writing when dictated to, my right hand—with which I was writing at the time—while making the lateral movements, would also be pulled in a twisting motion, lifting the pen off the paper every now and then. This would make the controlled rhythmic movement required for continuous writing very difficult. The intensity of this kept increasing as time went by, and when I reached about age fifteen writing more than a few words legibly had become almost a total impossibility. My older sister at that time would often write for me. For my letters I would write as best I could, then she would copy what she could read and I would dictate what she couldn't. Being a farm boy, the work I did comprised mainly chores and driving machinery and maintaining it. For this my motion disorder as yet was of very little hindrance.

By the time I reached the age of fifteen I had started to develop a twitch in my left leg at the knee. Walking, especially when I was tired or under any emotional stress, became progressively more difficult. By the time I reached age 25 I had also developed a spastic twitch at my right ankle. This developed into a pattern that would turn the right foot inward, also twisting it sideways so that when moving the right leg forward for the next step, my toe would often catch behind my heel. This would frequently cause me to stumble and also at times to fall. One thing that puzzled me, though, was that I still could run with a relatively smooth and unhindered stride. To this day a slow run when I am tired usually works better for me than walking.

At about age seventeen I started to notice a twitch in my neck. This would happen when I would be making a rotating type of movement like shovelling grain. This twitch in my neck kept on increasing in intensity, developing into a rotating type of pull on my head. The uncontrollable pull was always to the left. When I would try to hold it stable, anywhere from center to the right position, it would just pull back to the left just past center, where I could then hold it, but still with some difficulty. I could always at will move my head anywhere I wanted to, but as soon as I stopped it at any position from center to the right, it would always pull back, rotating it to the left. I had still some difficulty to even keep it there.

———————

Andre's description illustrates the progressive nature of certain types of dystonia, especially when symptoms appear early in life. The pattern of progression, however, was different for him than for others afflicted with generalized dystonia.

Al, who lives with his wife on an island in Washington State, ended his career as a naval officer prematurely, after several years of being virtually unable to speak. In recent years, he has recovered some of that ability, though his voice is raspy and uneven.

How long has your voice been affected?

From 1959 till 1992 I had no voice. It turned out that I was able to do some jobs without the speech. When I was on the ship I could generally squeeze out enough words to get my points across. But when I went to the ordinance supply office, most of my communication was by writing. At that time I couldn't even speak on the telephone. That reminds me of some of the other things that the psychiatrists used to do. They would have me say a lot of different words, and the words that I hung up on the most they figured that there was some emotional relationship. Actually, it's not emotional. There are some words the pronunciation of which is easier for anybody. Some words are harder to bring the cords together just in ordinary speech. I think it was these types of words that I had my hang-up on.

Al's form of dystonia is called *spasmodic dysphonia*, in which the tiny muscles in the larynx that control the vocal cords tighten uncontrollably and cause distorted speech. When these spasms occurred, before Al had been properly diagnosed and treated, the normal muscle modulations necessary to produce speech were stopped. He was essentially mute.

Deirdre is not only mute but incapacitated in nearly every other way except intellectually. I didn't meet or see her, but I talked with her father, Scott, who described the onset of her dystonia fully and poignantly.

Your daughter's symptoms began appearing very early in her life, is that right?

She was born in 1984—about four pounds, twelve ounces and she went to full term. As time went on she was doing fine. She had a sucking problem—feeding. But then around two years old she still wasn't walking yet or talking, so we were concerned and we had her evaluated at Northshore Hospital [on Long Island, New York]. And they said that she's delayed, you know, she may have some mental problem. One neurologist said that she would be retarded, which she's not at all.

Were they attributing this to some kind of birth defect?

Yes. But they didn't know what. And then as soon as we took her to the neurologist right after that she started walking and talking. But she was floppy so she was diagnosed as hypotonic. And she was always floppy and she was always a little behind, but nothing really drastic—maybe six months behind as she was going through nursery school—and they were a little concerned. And then her last year in nursery school, she was almost caught up. Her last year of nursery school she was five, they would say, "She's at four years, eight months." She was very close.

And then her foot started to curl, and then it just went away. And then her neck started to move like this—just back and forth—and then that went away. Then about five months later her neck started again, and it's been downhill ever since. Her neck was back like this [arches his neck back]. She couldn't walk. Then she got her walking back but it was very difficult for her to walk, and throughout the years she progressed to the point now where she can't walk. Her speech is affected by it. She has—you can't understand her—very few words like yes and no, whereas when she was three or four years old she had a very slight speech problem but you could understand her perfectly clearly. She's homebound now because she can't go to school.

———

Deirdre has generalized dystonia, in which nearly every muscle of her body is affected. Hers is one of the most extreme forms of dystonia.

By contrast, my dystonia is minor. The symptoms were first noticeable only when I wrote with my right hand. Several years ago, after I had become exclusively a left-hander for all my writing and typing, I wrote about the evolution of my writing difficulty in a journal:

"I first noticed my handwriting beginning to change—becoming smaller, more cramped. Since I am a teacher, I write all the time, so it was easy to conclude that something was wrong with muscles in my hand or arm. Over a two- or three-year period, the writer's cramp— that's what it felt like—increased so that writing with a pen or pencil for more than two or three minutes became extremely difficult, and the writing quality was deteriorating, becoming smaller and less legible as I struggled to sustain legibility while also writing reasonably fast. Typing, too, became difficult—my right elbow rising beyond the normal typing angle, the whole arm tending toward contortion. I would try consciously to relax, to will the tension away, but without more than momentary success."

———

The term *writer's cramp* applies to the kind of dystonia I have, although the muscle tension seems to originate in the shoulder and affects the whole arm. The act of writing, which requires acute small-muscle coordination, is the most severely affected; the dystonia is also apparent in the abnormal swing of my arm as I walk. Aside from some muscular soreness that arises from the almost constant tensing of the shoulder muscles, there is no pain.

When you have misbehaving muscles or muscular soreness that won't go away—and you know it's not just because of strenuous activity—you have to wonder what might be the cause. When you're having continual difficulty in speaking and you know it's not just a sore throat, how do you try to explain it? If you're crossing a busy street or driving your car and your eyes force themselves shut, what do you suspect is happening? If, as happened with Deirdre, dystonia knocks you flat—makes you a complete invalid—will not you, or your parents, scour the medical community to find an answer?

Most Americans live with an expectation that physical ailments have knowable causes, even if diseases like cancer and AIDS are not yet fully explained. So, when muscles go berserk, as they do in dystonia, a typical reaction is to go in search of a cause. Unlike Peter, however, whose physician-father was fully prepared to explain his symptoms to him, most people who experience symptoms of dystonia go on long, often disappointing, searches for a correct diagnosis.

Chapter 3

Searching for a Diagnosis

Although descriptions of dystonia have appeared in medical literature since the early part of this century, getting an accurate and prompt diagnosis has been more unusual than typical for many people. The usual clinical tests come up negative, so doctors are often as mystified as the patient.

Candace went for several years without a correct diagnosis—critical years because she was adolescent.

What do you remember about trying to get a good medical explanation for your symptoms?

My parents started taking me to doctors when I was about twelve years old. My background was that I was the fifth child out of six. I came from an alcoholic family so I really didn't get the attention I needed, and I compensated with it because I was very strong. At nine years I could go the whole day. I just got tired in the later afternoon. My school work was affected from it. I was left back in third grade. At the time they thought it was just a learning disability, but now, as I've researched it, it was definitely the dystonia. But when they did start taking me to the doctors, I was first diagnosed with a drop foot, and they gave me exercises to do and just said that the muscles in the calf and the front of the leg needed to be built up, and nothing worked.

And then they took me to neurologists, and they did EMGs [electromyograms] and nerve conductor tests and nothing showed. My leg was fine. My hips were fine. Everything was functioning.

Did they act mystified?

No, not at all. They just thought I was dumb. One did act mystified, but it really wasn't something he wanted to pursue ... had a lazy leg that ... I had a drop foot. If I did exercises, the leg would get better.

Was anybody implying or saying that maybe you were faking this?

Oh, yes. Every doctor said that I was faking it. Every doctor said that "she has no reason to be acting like this." The last doctor I went to ... I'll never forget it. I was sixteen years old. He put me on the table and he must have stuck at least 100 needles up and down my legs, trying to prove to me that there was nothing wrong. My mother was out in the waiting room, and I was just hysterical 'cause he took these needles that had to be at least six or seven inches long and made sure that he got to the nerve, and then he moved the needle around. He showed me on the monitor that there was nerve activity. When I got out of the office I said to my mother, "I'm not doing this anymore."

————

Al, whose speech became impaired when he was a naval officer, heard from Navy physicians that his problem might be mental.

What was your experience in getting a diagnosis about your difficulty with speaking?

When I first experienced the spasmodic dysphonia in 1959, the doctors were all concerned that it was psychiatric, so I was referred to psychiatrists and I continued to see psychiatrists and they did their thing to work on my mind. They had very little previous experience with this condition. I never did see a neurologist. Perhaps a neurologist would have recognized the symptoms. I first went to a throat specialist. He looked at my throat and had me take cough medicine. I went to Bethesda, and he finally decided he couldn't do any good and that's when they referred me to psychiatrists. I continued to see psychiatrists from 1959 until 1979. It was the only game in town. To tell the truth, when I was getting the psychiatric treatment I didn't tell anybody except my wife that I was going to a psychiatrist. I still have hang-ups about that. I think the stigma is worse for having been treated psychiatrically than for having dystonia.

One psychiatrist put me on truth serum—something like laughing gas, nitrous oxide—and tried to question me back to my youth and find out if I'd had any trauma. I thought it was ridiculous, but it was still the only game in town so I didn't give it up. But I think the point when I finally decided it was completely ridiculous was when the last psychiatrist—the one from the Veterans Hospital—when I'd go to my car, would have me scream at the top of my lungs for the entire trip. I'd leave here [Seattle] and drive to Tacoma and scream. Apparently, that was supposed to relieve emotional tension.

Though Al has, of course, completely rejected the diagnosis that his disorder might have a psychiatric origin, he still retains some of the hurt. That feeling is shared by many other dystonia patients whose supposed mentors in the medical community have made them feel degrees of guilt about their symptoms. While a psychiatric disorder is not the fault of the individual, the supposed connection between emotional trauma and lost muscle control is at best confusing to the patient and at worst an additional burden of disability and hopelessness.

This conclusion is shared by Donald Calne and A.E. Lang, Canadian neurologists specializing in dystonia: "It is distressing for patients with an organic disease to be told, incorrectly, that the disease is in their mind, and that they can exert control over it by changing their mental attitude. In the case of children, it is equally upsetting for the parents to be saddled with the implied responsibility of having failed in some way to give their offspring whatever was required for normal development. In such circumstances, the diagnosis of organic dystonia is generally accepted with relief because neither the patient nor their family can be regarded as blameworthy." (The source for this statement and for medical information later in this chapter is articles by Donald B. Calne, A.E. Lang, and Stanley Fahn in **Advances in Neurology, Vol. 50: Dystonia 2**, Raven Press, 1988.)

James, who lives alone in an apartment in the Puget Sound region of Washington State, spends most of his time in a wheelchair. He only fairly recently found out the nature of a progressive disability that has afflicted him since childhood.

Who told you that you have dystonia?

It wasn't until I came up here [to Washington] five years ago. I didn't know I had dystonia from the time of birth till I was 35 years old. I didn't know what it was. My mother's a nurse, and they came down to California where I was at. She came and got me first. At that point, I was crawling around. I had been walking on the top of my feet for almost four years. I had lost a home to medical bills because they couldn't figure out what was wrong with me. They thought it was MS [multiple sclerosis] but it didn't qualify—the odd movements, the being tired, and the constricting in my muscles, and the deterioration in the muscles made them believe ... and I also at that time had broken my back. I'd had a fusion done in 1978. The right leg turned so the foot was backwards and they couldn't get it to come around forward. Whenever I would start to walk at all, it would turn itself upside down.

I'd gotten so tired of being told I was nuts, I was crazy, it was all in my head. Doctors and family were telling me that—the people I would see that I thought would know what was wrong. They just said, "Well, we don't know what it is. It must be in your head." After losing a home because of the medical bills, I just stopped going to any type of medical practice whatsoever and just said, "To hell with it." I crawled around on my hands and knees or I walked on the top of my feet for quite a while—extremely painful—which then led me to even use more drugs. But after so many years of being told that you're just making it up, even in the back of my own head it was kinda like you think that that's the way it is.

It's still hard for me today to realize I have dystonia. It's just been put in there so deeply, for so long. It's hard for me to remember that I'm supposed to lay down and rest, I'm not supposed to get up and do this. It's always been one where if I willed it, it didn't matter what I had to do, I would do it. If I had to crawl to something or whatever, I did whatever I had to do to do it. I was very headstrong. I just said, "The hell with it."

I finally saw a rehabilitation neurologist here in Tacoma. At that point I had braces on my legs and the Canadian canes. They thought for about a year in California that the only thing it could be is MS with complications from the spine, but it wasn't that bad, and it wouldn't progress. When I came up here, I wanted to find out what can I do because my legs had shrunk in size to almost what my arms are now from atrophying. The only way I could get around was to try and walk, and it was like walking like a ballerina for the first three or four steps. Then I was walking on the tops and it hurt like hell. So I just crawled. As you can see, I still keep my kneepads around. I'd just crawl where I had to go and pull myself up and do it that way.

I had fought the feeling of suicide for many years, had made many attempts because I hurt all the time. The only way not to hurt was to take the strong pain killers and speed so that I could keep going. And in doing so it made the dystonia worse because it affected the same area of the brain. So I was doing more damage to myself, but yet everybody told me that there was nothing wrong with me. So I figured, well, if I just do this stuff at least I can make a living a little bit, which ended up going through being married twice, losing a home. When I came out of the hospital in '78, my wife had left.

When the Tacoma neurologist said *dystonia***, had you ever heard the word before?**

Never.

What did he say about dystonia and how you fitted into that diagnosis?

He had me get up and walk, using the Canadian canes, down the hallway and back. Then he had me sit down again and he told me about the word dystonia. He said that for a long time it was thought just to be within a certain "tribe" of Jewish people where he had come from. But that when my feet turned in as I tried to walk, my posture— the way I twisted—that it could very possibly be dystonia and that dystonia was very hard to know what it was because there was no specific test.

He said it was pretty much limited to Ashkenazi Jews but you fitted the description?

Well, I laughed at him because I told him, I said, "A lot of the doctors that have seen me have asked me if I'm Jewish. I thought they were joking with me that I was Jewish." He told me a little bit about it. He told me that it was in the brain, that it could have been brought on by many things. There were tests that he wanted me to take. They did the MRI, the CT scan, the one that they hook up the electrodes to your eyes and so on and you see different patterns and so on. After looking at the results, the doctor said, "You have dystonia and you have full-body or generalized ... that great big word ... musculorum deformans." I asked him, "Why is it called that?" He said, "It deforms your muscle." He says part of them are going to contract and contract and I said, "Is that where the pain comes from?"

―――――――

The term *musculorum deformans* that James quoted is seldom used now in the medical community, though it has long-standing usage. These Latin words refer to altered muscle tone and subsequent postural deformities. Because dystonia is not a disease of the muscles, the term has generally been replaced by the terms *idiopathic torsion dystonia, primary dystonia,* and *generalized dystonia.* Other terms (listed at the end of this chapter) specify each type of secondary dystonia.

Elena, a Canadian graduate student at the time her neck began to behave strangely, sought out her general practitioner.
Who finally diagnosed your dystonia?
Well, it was about four months between the first symptoms and the skiing accident, and I did go to my G.P. [general practitioner] once during that time. She told me that it must be nerves. That's what they usually do.

After she had made a careful assessment of your temperament?

Yeah. [laughs] Well, actually, I was in university and I was getting a scholarship. I was going to be studying overseas for my final year, and so there was a lot of pressure on me to perform. I was working to support myself at the same time. There was actually a phenomenal amount of pressure. My sister was quite ill. She'd had cranial surgery twice during that year so there was a lot going on. That explanation made sense to me, too, at the time. I thought, "Well, you know, that would kind of fit. I really do have an awful lot of stress." But then after the skiing accident, it didn't make sense any more. The stress didn't fit it because it was just getting worse and worse. I went to my G.P. actually nine times during that year—over a one-year period—because it was getting worse quickly, and she wasn't doing anything.

Did she say she'd ever seen anything like it?

No. As a matter of fact what she diagnosed it as was wry neck. She sent me to physiotherapy, which was actually the best thing she could have done because I went to a sports clinic where they did massage, and the massage was absolutely wonderful and really calmed some of those symptoms down. But it took a year before I was diagnosed with dystonia. I was diagnosed by an internist in a dinky, little hospital in a small town in southern Ontario.

Did that internist call it *dystonia*?

I think he said spasmodic torticollis. I don't think he said dystonia. I don't know whether I heard the name used.

That's rather common.

Yeah. I don't think I heard dystonia until I saw a neurologist. So I ended up going to two different neurologists.

Spasmodic torticollis is a term more firmly established in certain portions of the medical community than the more general term *dystonia*, probably because the word *torticollis* (for *twisted neck*) has a longer history of use. Since the symptom of a twisted neck can result from several causes other than neurological, not tying spasmodic torticollis to the broader term *dystonia* may fail to lead to a correct diagnosis.

Marjorie, who lives in Seattle, heard the term *spasmodic torticollis* over thirty years ago, though it took a long time to go any further than knowing the term for what she had.

How and when did you get accurate information about what was wrong with your neck?

At the age of 24, I was working at a job and at that time my head started to turn to the left. It seemed to be gradual. This one girl at work said, "I have a good osteopathic physician." So I went to see him. He told me immediately it was spasmodic torticollis. This was over thirty years ago. He never talked about dystonia. He just said, "You have spasmodic torticollis." I didn't know what it was—whether it was mental or physical.

So just throughout the years I'd always be going to different doctors. One doctor treated it. He did manipulation and everything on it, which just didn't help. In discussing why I had this condition, he mentioned stress. He said I was in a very bad marriage—later on. I think at that time they thought it was more emotional because they would give you different tranquilizers and medication. I myself thought it was mental. There were so many different things that went on. At one time, he put me in the hospital. I was just laying almost chained in the bed. It was to hold you straight. I was in there for a number of days. And then he put me under hypnosis and took me all the way back to my childhood, thinking that it was an emotional thing.

It was soon after I was diagnosed, that same year, that I was pregnant. It sort of left me at that time. When I was pregnant, it was like you were in remission. And then it would start up again.

I think the worst time was when my head went to one side for six months and just stayed in a fixed position. You couldn't move your head at all. I went to one doctor who did a lot of massage and things like that. He gave me a lot of shots and I don't know what they were. I'd get it for a minute or so that my head would go straight. Then gradually it started coming back. It still would pull to one side, but at least I got it where it was halfway straight. That in itself was an accomplishment. For six months it never moved. So it was difficult.

Helen, also a resident of Washington State, had an experience similar to Marjorie's. The process of trying to get a diagnosis also involved her in treatments that were largely irrelevant to the condition, though some of them brought temporary relief from the pain of muscular tension.

What were the earliest symptoms of dystonia for you?

Actually it was a problem of hanging on to the pen when I was writing. My hand didn't cramp up but it felt as if I didn't have the strength to hang on to the pen. Actually what I guess it was doing was rolling off the ends of my fingers.

That was how long ago?

That was five years ago—about five and a half years ago.

When did you know, then, that you had an affliction that was called dystonia?

Actually I didn't know that until probably this spring [1993]. I had a problem with my hand that started about five and a half years ago, and I began to have problems with my head tipping just sort of very gently to the right. That began I think about ... almost three years ago.

Not much pain though?

No, not at that time. I really didn't have too much pain until about two years ago. It was mostly just the tipping and it didn't do it all the time and then it would also tilt to the left and up or twist to the left and up. It probably was about two or two-and-a-half years ago that it started to be uncomfortable and then just ... I didn't really know what it was or what was going on and it just got worse and worse. As far as my hand ... I did see a number of different neurologists and whatnot and they thought that ... we did some testing for carpal tunnel and I had that a couple times—surgery—and it didn't make any difference. I was treated for tendonitis. I took time off from work. The tendonitis did clear up, but nothing improved in my hand. My head kept getting worse. Maybe last fall I did see a doctor. I saw a physiatrist and he said, "Well, you have torticollis." They tried some injections. I can't remember what it is, but it's something they injected into the muscle—not something you would get if you had work done on your teeth but a similar idea—that it was going to deaden the muscle for a certain length of time. What they were working on was the fact that it was in a spasm, so they thought, if they did that, that when the muscle recovered, it would not have a memory of being in spasm and so my head would be fine. We tried that and that didn't work.

What kind of a doctor was that?

It was a physiatrist. It's physical medicine—a rehabilitation specialist. So we tried that two different times, and it didn't make any difference. Then he said, "Well, you have torticollis." I said, "I don't know what that is." He said, "It's what your neck is doing, and your muscles are in spasm." He suggested that I might want to try a chiropractor to see if that made any difference. He also said, "If you want, you could try acupuncture." So I tried all of those. I did get a little relief with the chiropractor at first, but I think that was because I was having ... I didn't know this but it was actually pinched nerves and some of the manipulation he did relieved some of the pain in my arm and my fingers that were going numb. But at first I went once a week, then I found I was almost having to go every other day if I was going to have any relief, so I decided it wasn't effective in the long term. With physical therapy, again it would give me some relief, particularly across my muscles in my back ... that was just the secondary spasming or whatnot that was going on. And again at first that would last for maybe a week and then I'd leave the office and by the time I was in the car everything was painful again.

———————

Even in a small city in Eastern Washington, more than thirty years ago, it was possible at least to avoid a misleading diagnosis, as Ted attested.

What were your first symptoms? What were you noticing in the 1960s?

At that time it was just more like a tremor. My head was like that [briefly demonstrates the way his head used to shake] all the time. On a real bad day it would come over and almost lock on the shoulder. I could cure that by touching my chin with one finger, and this is really the first way of recognizing torticollis. But the doctor over there in Richland [in eastern Washington, near the Hanford Nuclear Reservation] said, "Yeah, I know what you got. You've got spasmodic torticollis."

That doctor was a neurologist?

Yeah, and supposed to be real good. "We don't know what cures it. We don't know much about it, but the best thing for you to do is go back to your family physician and then start working from there."

Ted spent the next several years trying various treatments, with varying success, but, unlike many others, he avoided a misleading or long-delayed diagnosis.

Andre—whose symptoms appeared in his hand, foot, and neck—doesn't remember who first gave a name to his disability, but one term reverberated for many years: *cerebral palsy*. Indeed, the symptoms of cerebral palsy and dystonia can seem similar and both disabilities stem from dysfunctions in the brain. It was after several years of trying "brain patterning" exercises said to help cerebral-palsied individuals—many repetitions of the desired movement patterns in arms and legs—that Andre eventually got an accurate diagnosis. That was in 1985, when he was in his 50s. The diagnosis offered little hope, though.

What did your doctor tell you?

He said that as yet very little was known about dystonia and that there was as yet nothing developed for treatment of the disorder. The only thing he knew that was of any value was a lot of walking for a relaxing exercise.

———————

That neurologist's information was inaccurate or incomplete, though it was apparently typical. Dystonia was being treated in 1985 in some movement-disorder centers, but these treatments had not become widely known among neurologists and certainly not among general practitioners.

Because dystonia symptoms are so varied—some of them resembling symptoms of other disorders—and because the usual tests do not lead to an accurate diagnosis, many patients go from one medical office to another. In a place such as New York City, however, the likelihood of getting an accurate diagnosis has for several years been greater than in many other parts of the country. Louise, who lives in Queens, near Manhattan, is an example of one dystonia patient who didn't have to wait long for her diagnosis.

When do you remember, then, saying, "Can we do something about this?"

Well, it wasn't me. I remember ... what happened was ... after fifth grade my parents sent me away to sleepaway camp, and it was an eight-week camp. What had happened that made them realize that something was wrong was they saw the way I was walking when they sent me off to camp that summer. And then they came up to visit one time—like parents' visiting day—and then they saw me eight weeks later when I came home, and they realized that there was a big difference between the way I was walking when I left for camp and the way I was walking when I came home. And I think that that's what made my parents realize that something was wrong and they needed to start figuring out what was happening to me. So I don't remember saying, "Mom, we have to do something about this." I just remember my parents thinking that they should do something about it, try and figure out what was going on.

So what did they do?

They started taking me to all kinds of doctors. We went to ... not an orthopedist ... I think maybe it was an orthopedist—bone doctor. And he didn't know what was wrong and he suggested that we go to a neurologist. We went to a neurologist at LIJ—Long Island Jewish Hospital—and she was the person who diagnosed me. She had just recently finished her training and stuff so she wanted to be sure so she sent us to the person who was her teacher or supervisor. He saw me and he confirmed it and then my parents wanted another opinion so they took me to a third neurologist and he confirmed it. He said, "Yes, she has dystonia."

―――――――

For Louise's mother, though, the route to a diagnosis seemed a little different.

Why did you decide to take Louise to see a neurologist?

The only reason we went to a neurologist was because I took her to many doctors and she used to cry at night, "Mommy, I ... everything's pulling, everything's pulling." I took her to the pediatrician: "It's growing pains, it's growing pains." I took her to so many places. I took her to the orthopedist, and he said, "I don't know what the hell it is, but I have kids and if this were my kid I would take her to a neurologist." That's just how it came about.

Now, in retrospect, are you surprised that he recognized it right away?

No, because he said he had about five or six other patients, and actually that's what we were looking for. We were looking for a doctor who had treated other patients. The doctor at LIJ [Long Island Jewish Hospital] had never seen a dystonic. She remembered her notes when she went to medical school. She had come across these things. She spent three hours testing our daughter with another doctor, and from her notes and discussing this with the other doctor she decided that this was dystonia.

She ruled out other possibilities?
That's right.

————

Louise's mother pointed out that the LIJ doctor had never seen a person with dystonia symptoms, but before reaching a tentative conclusion she ruled out other possibilities. This is exactly the process that physicians must use in arriving at a diagnosis of dystonia. First, they apply several tests to determine what **isn't** causing the symptoms. Then, they observe the patient's movements carefully and take a history of his or her symptoms to see whether this patient's condition matches medical descriptions of one of the forms of dystonia.

The physician who is usually best able to diagnose dystonia correctly is a neurologist, because dystonia is a disorder centered in the brain. Nerve impulses mediated in the basal ganglia, a deep relay station in the brain, overstimulate muscles. The result of too much nerve activity is a tensing or spasming of the affected muscle. Exactly why the nerves start acting this way is unknown.

Because so much is unknown about the physiology of dystonia, the most knowledgeable neurologists presently suggest that we call dystonia a **syndrome**—a group of symptoms that are characteristic of the disease or disorder they call dystonia. Specifically, they say that dystonia "is a syndrome of sustained muscle contractions, frequently causing twisting and repetitive movements, or abnormal postures." (Fahn in **Advances in Neurology, Vol. 50: Dystonia 2**)

With this as the broad definition, neurologists try to fit their observations of a patient's movements and medical history into one of several classifications.

Dystonia: The Disease That Distorts

The following questions and tentative con-
clusions suggest the process of figuring out what
the problem is.

Age at appearance of symptoms

At what age did the patient start noticing abnormal muscle behavior:
childhood (up to 12 years),
adolescence (13-20 years), or adulthood?
Tentative conclusion: The
younger the patient, the
more likely it is that the
dystonia is idiopathic or
primary.

Probable cause

Is there a history of dystonia in the
patient's family?
Tentative conclusion: If so, the
patient's disorder may
be hereditary (that is,
genetic). This is idio-
pathic or primary
dystonia. If not, a ge-
netic cause can not be
ruled out, though the
cause may lie else-
where.
Does the patient have a history of one
of several degenerative, neurological
disorders, such as, Wilson's disease,
Leigh's disease, Fahr's disease, or
Huntington's disease?

Tentative conclusion: If so,
    damage may have oc-
    curred in the basal gan-
    glia. The diagnosis may
    be secondary dystonia.
Has the patient had some type of brain
injury not associated with degeneration of brain cells, such as, birth injury, brain tumor, head trauma, en-
cephalitis, drugs?
Tentative conclusion: If so,
    damage may have oc-
    curred in the basal gan-
    glia. The diagnosis may
    be secondary dystonia.

<u>Part(s) of body affected</u>
    Is a single body part affected, such
as, eyelids, mouth, larynx, neck, arm?
Tentative conclusion: If so,
    this may be a focal
    dystonia, which may
    remain in this body part
    or may spread to other
    parts of the body.
Do the dystonic symptoms affect two
or more contiguous body parts, such
as, head and neck, neck and trunk, leg
and trunk?
Tentative conclusion: If so,
    this may be segmental
    dystonia, which may
    represent the spreading
    of a focal dystonia.

Are one or both legs, as well as some other region of the body, affected? Tentative conclusion: If so, this may be generalized dystonia.

Are two or more noncontiguous body parts affected, such as left arm and right leg, or one leg and the neck? Tentative conclusion: If so, this may be multifocal dystonia.

Is one-half of the body affected, for example, leg and arm on same side; leg, arm, and face on same side? Tentative conclusion: If so, this may be hemi-dystonia, a form that is almost always second-ary rather than primary.

When the neurologist has arrived at a diag-nosis, he or she may use still other terms to label the specific form of dystonia, particularly the fo-cal dystonias. They include the following:

term	symptom(s)
blepharospasm [BLEFF - uh - ro - spazm]	eyelids close uncontrollably
cervical dystonia [SURR - vih - kuhl, or surr- VY - kuhl]	neck muscles twist neck to either side; neck may pull, turn or jerk; shoulder on one side may rise
spasmodic torticollis [spaz - MOD -ik tor - tih - KOHL - uhs]	same as symptoms for cervical dystonia
antecollis (form of cervical dystonia) [AN - tee - kohl - uhs]	neck muscles twist forward
retrocollis (form of cervical dystonia) [RET - ro - kohl - uhs]	neck muscles twist backward
cranial dystonia [KRAYN - ee- uhl diss - TOHN - ee- uh]	two or more parts of the head are affected (such as, eyes and mouth)
spasmodic dysphonia [spaz - MOD -ik diss - TOHN - ee- uh]	vocal cords draw tightly together or pull apart, resulting in distorted speech
laryngeal dystonia [lar - RIN - gee - uhl diss - TOHN - ee- uh]	same as symptoms for spasmodic dysphonia

Dystonia: The Disease That Distorts

term	symptom(s)
writer's cramp	muscles of hand or fingers cramp during writing
musician's cramp	muscles of hand or fingers cramp when the individual plays a stringed instrument or the piano, for example
Meige's syndrome [MAY - zhuz SIN - drohm]	muscles of lower face irregularly pull, or jaw muscles pull mouth open or closed
orofacial-buccal dystonia [AW - ro - FAY - shuhl BUCK - uhl diss - TOHN - ee - uh]	same as symptoms for Meige's syndrome
Segawa's dystonia [seg - AH - wuhz diss - TOHN - ee- uh]	muscles in several parts of body become mildly rigid and movements awkward
dopa-responsive dystonia [DOH -puh ree - SPON- sihv diss - TOHN - ee- uh]	same as symptoms for Segawa's dystonia

When a neurologist finally uses one of these terms and explains, the best he or she can, the nature of the disorder, patients often move to another plane of acceptance. The mysterious symptoms now have a name. Having a label, validated by the medical community, offers at least a glimmer of understanding and sparks a hope for relief from the spasms of the distorted muscle.

Chapter 4

Searching for a Treatment

Medical science cannot presently offer a cure for dystonia; instead, doctors and their patients can only search for something that might relieve symptoms. This search often leads through an array of drugs: muscle-relaxants, tranquilizers, anti-convulsants, anti-psychotics, and anti-cholinergics (drugs that block nerve impulses). More recently, a unique kind of injection directly into affected muscles has offered temporary relief from spasming muscles. And brain or muscle-denervation surgery has also seemed a reasonable choice in some cases. Each case of dystonia, though, is different, so the search for a suitable treatment is likely to be lengthy and, in a number of cases, may ultimately be less than satisfactory.

Peter, the 13-year-old whose physician father could monitor the effects of the various drugs he tried, described his search as a kind of experiment.

Tell me about your recent experience with medications.

We were going on different medicines and when they didn't work, we, you know, lowered them or took them completely off and tried different medicines. And so what seemed to happen was after a while, even without any medicine, you know, in the morning I'd walk bad and at 3 o'clock I'd walk fine and no one would notice anything and 7 o'clock or when I'd get tired it comes back again. It seems, if I get bad and we raise my medicine, it takes at least a week to two weeks before anything happens, and sometimes after two weeks it gets bad and we're like, "I don't know. Should we change it again?" And then three days later it's fine, so we're like, "Oh, we might as well keep the medicine where we are" and four days later it's bad.

Right now you're in a good period, then, is that right?

Right now, yeah, I'm in a good period.

When you say "change the medicine," do you mean to go to a different medicine or increase the dose of the one you've been taking?

Increase the dosage, lower it, take it off, try new medicine, all that.

You're still experimenting with that all the time?

Yes.

Are you taking the same ones your brother is?

Yeah, I'm taking two of his three. The two I'm taking are Baclofen [muscle-relaxant] and Artane [anti-cholinergic].

What's the dose now, do you know?

Uhhh, all I know is I take five Artane and two Baclofen four times a day.

What other effects do you notice besides some improvement?

Ahhh, sometimes my legs get better and my hands get worse, like when I first started to get dystonia bad in my hands, it was mostly in my right hand, so I worked hard and I switched to my left hand, and lately it's been hard for my left hand so I'm back to my right hand. It's difficult, so it gets switching and worse and better and better and worse. Sometimes even if I'm in a good walking period, if I walk down a hall with a lot of people around me, I walk poorly versus if I'm just walking down an empty hall with no one around me I can walk fine. Sometimes if I'm walking down the hall alone and someone I don't know is walking up at me, that's when I get nervous, and so I get nervous because I'm like "What's this person gonna think?" and that's when I get bad. I try and stay unnervous so that my symptoms don't show as badly.

———————

Robert, a 12-year-old half-reclined on a table when I interviewed him, having arrived in a wheelchair pushed by his father. As we talked, muscles twitched in his arms and legs and his speech was often difficult to understand because of facial spasms. His terse answers to my questions, however, seemed unrelated to his spasms. He, too, is in a decidedly experimental period so far as medications are concerned.

Have you tried any kind of pills?
Oh, yeah.
What? Tell me about that.
They experiment in drugs on me. The BOTOX [injection of botulinum toxin] is to see

what ... it's a drug that they're seeing what it'll do, and I've been on a lot of different medicines.

Do you remember the names?

There was Tegretol [anti-convulsant]...

Artane [anti-cholinergic]?

Yeah. The ones now are Cogentin [benztropine, an agent which annuls or antagonizes a part of the autonomic nervous system], TBZ [tetrabenazine, a tranquilizer], lorazepam [anti-anxiety] ...

You're taking all of those now?

Yeah.

Do you think they help?

Yeah.

What do they do?

They relax my muscles.

How do you know they do?

You feel it.

If you stopped taking the drugs, would you be different?

Yes.

Very different?

Yes.

How different?

I would be thrashing.

Thrashing. Both arms and both legs and your neck?

Yeah.

So when you have the medication and the BOTOX [botulinum toxin], you say you're pretty good?

Yes.

You can do most things?
Yes.
So it sounds to me as though you're not too unhappy about this.
Yeeuh.
No special reason to be unhappy?
I've coped with it so it doesn't bother me anymore.
You don't think about it much?
No.

———

Melinda—who has braces on her hands, arms, and legs to partially control her otherwise erratic movements—was about 20 years old when she first noticed the symptoms of generalized dystonia. From then on, after years of seeking a proper diagnosis, she has tried numerous medications. She now takes several each day and manages, most of the time, to report for work five days a week in a large government office in Queens.

What led to your getting the medications you needed to gain some control over your movement?

I made the rounds of all of the major doctors and hospitals in the area. I finally came across a doctor, after taking one look at me and five minutes figuring out what I had—that I had dystonia. That was a doctor up at Mt. Sinai [in New York City].

A neurologist?

A neurologist, yeah. He was head of the department up there. After just taking a look, he figured out what it was. So they tried me on various medications.

By the way, did he label it further—a specific type of dystonia?

No, at that time they didn't. See, my stuff progressed very slowly. First it started with the head tremor that would come and go, then eventually it just came and it wouldn't go anywhere. It stayed around for a long time. I then developed problems with the right arm. The reason I wear the braces is my arms are literally flying all over the place without them on. Basically what the braces do is they control the movement enough that I can use ... pretty much use the arms.

Does it now appear that it's generalized dystonia?

Yeah. For me the last thing that went was the legs. Some people it's the first. For me it was...

Yours was the later onset?

Mine was considered adult onset. I was either 20 or 21 when it was first discovered ... in that time span. Over the years it's progressed, I've been in and out of a wheelchair. I just came out of a chair again. It forced me to stop working for two years and go on disability because I mean the whole body really went. Even now I still have a lot of problems. I'm on a tremendous amount of medication.

Do you have a combination of medications that seems to work fairly well now?

Ummm. Kind of. I'm still having ...

Compared to how bad it might have been or has been?

There's not as much as ... there's more than I've had in a while but not as much as I would like to have. I'm still having a very big problem with getting the spasticity under control in the arms. The legs seem to have quieted down a little but the arms are really still ...

What are the medications now?

I'm on Artane [anti-cholinergic], reserpine [anti-hypertensive], Clozaril [anti-psychotic], ephedrine [decongestant], and Baclofen [muscle-relaxant].

That's quite a combination. High dosages?

Yeah. My Artane ... I can't tolerate a whole lot ... my Artane is about 20 milligrams right now. It varies. One of them I think I'm on like 100 milligrams a day. The others I don't even know. After a while you lose track. You just know how many pills you're taking.

You must have noticed some side-effects.

Yeah. The drug that causes me the most problem is the Artane. I have trouble speaking. I know what I want to say, but my head starts running faster than my mouth can keep up with. A lot of times I'll have to just kind of stop and regroup and start all over again.

Has it affected memory?

Not that much. I don't think I'm taking a high enough dosage for me to ... but sometimes you know you get that ... it's like you're dull, like you're not completely sharp. Someone might say something and there's a slight delay in processing time from the time you actually hear it and comprehend and when it's said. Everybody knows about the dry mouth. I live with my bottle of water, sitting and drinking during the day.

———————

Melinda's reference to unpleasant—or worse—side-effects echoes a common complaint of people who are attempting to control dystonia symptoms with medication. Their constant search is for a balance between symptomatic treatment and loss of other valued capacities, such as accurate memory and general alertness.

Howard, a 63-year-old man living alone in New York City, explained his unfortunate experience with a medication that brings relief for some dystonia patients but was making his life appreciably worse.

Are the symptoms in the upper part of your body painful at all?

Oh, yeah. The amount of pain ... well, you can see I'm sweating [The interview took place on a cool, rainy day in a room where the temperature was less than 70 degrees.] The choice is whether or not to be doped up and in bed all the time or awake and in pain. That's all there is to it. Those are the options. Right now I'm off of everything. The little amount of Klonopin [anti-anxiety] I'd been taking maybe about three weeks ago, and I can feel it but I think that it might be a cycle ... I might have more spasms now and less a little later if I wait to get the drug cleaned out.

What was the Klonopin doing that you didn't like?

Well, I only took a half a milligram, but it just pretty much anesthetized me—just at the low-

56

est level, a half a milligram per diem. If I go back on it I can really feel it, even that minor amount, and yet that's the lightest dose.

Does it decrease the spasms at all?

It just puts me to sleep. It may decrease the spasms, but it just makes me very lethargic and I just want to be in bed all the time.

Sleeping eighteen hours a day, then, when you're on that?

Just about. I go to bed at four, five, six o'clock, I watch television and fall asleep for awhile. I'll wake up and then get out of bed at twelve noon the next day. A tremendous amount of time in bed. And then sometimes I go right through—have no desire to get up. Get up, fix something to eat, at three o'clock be back in bed. Even now it's a tendency I have—not really to be too responsive to any hour for getting up.

Does Tylenol or aspirin provide any relief?

No. Well, aspirin will settle my gut and that's about all, and there's a lot of what seem to be spasms down there.

So you're having digestion difficulty too?

Well, I can eat nails, but I seem to have a tough time with gas and cramps and things like that. Sometimes I have a very sore stomach or gut. My doctor seems to think it's a result of all the tension.

Sometimes, medication produces a stunning, positive result, as in the case of Candace. Accustomed since childhood to being a klutz, unable to control her "drop foot" and often losing her balance, she had an almost immediate disappearance of symptoms when she started taking the proper medication.

Describe how the medication affected you.

I had my son and six weeks later I went to see Dr. Fahn [a neurologist who specializes in movement disorders at Columbia University]. I must have been there for six or seven hours. He finally said, "You have dystonia. We have to put you in the hospital to do some tests ..." They had said to me, "If we can help you with the type of dystonia you have, either the medicine will work or it won't work." So I went into the hospital like three or four days after that, and they did a complete spinal tap, MRI, and they found that in my spinal fluid ... normal people have between fifty and seventy-five of a normal dopamine level ... I had eight. So they immediately started me on Sinemet [also called levadopa, which the body transforms into dopamine], and I walked out of the hospital normal. I just could not believe it. I must have done the stairs a hundred times. I went to the supermarket every day, walking up and down the aisles with the basket, and so proud of myself 'cause one leg would go in front of the other. I went dancing. I went running. And what happened was I pulled on the muscles in my upper body. I didn't give my body enough time to get used to the new way of walking.

Thinking your body was in better shape?

I just thought, "Wow. I'm just gonna do this just in case someone takes it away from me." So I just did everything, and what happened was I pulled all the muscles in my ribcage, and my right arm locked. It would not move . . . I'm on Sinemet. I take 3/4 of a tablet every day . . . from the time I first started with the symptoms to the time I was completely diagnosed and on medicine was twenty-five years.

Candace's dystonia proved to be "dopa-responsive." That is, her dystonia symptoms were caused by too little naturally produced dopamine in her brain. By taking a medication that boosts the supply of dopamine, she no longer experiences the symptoms of dystonia.

For Louise, who also began having dystonia symptoms during childhood, a different kind of medication gave relief that appeared to be equal to that experienced by Candace.

What combination of medications finally worked for you?

Once my parents found Dr. Barrett [a neurologist] he started me on medication—taking Artane [anti-cholinergic]. And then over the years it has changed. I've always been on Artane <u>and</u> something else. The something else has changed over the years, but the Artane has been the same— different dosage levels but I've been on Artane since I was about ten or eleven years old [She was about twenty-five at the time of the interview]. It helps. [laughs]

Many people speak about side-effects they don't like with Artane. Haven't you noticed any?

The first couple years I got cotton mouth. My mouth dried up. I don't really notice that anymore. I do notice, however, that they say some-times it can affect your memory. And I find that I forget things very quickly. People will tell me their name and if I don't use their name in something like saying, "Hello, Mr. So-and-so," I will forget their name.

I'd say you pass for normal on that.

Other things, too, just ... walking out of a store and leaving my package on the thing. It seems to me or at least I feel it happens more often than it should. And sometimes I feel like I'm walking around in a fog. It does ... sometimes I do feel like there is something that is clouding my ...

How does that affect your library work? Or maybe you don't want to say.

It doesn't really affect my library work. I've learned to get around it. I make notes for myself constantly and I'm always walking around ... I have a clipboard like this ... and I'm constantly walking around with reminders of "Call back so-and-so" or "Take care of this" or "Take care of that" and I mean if I ever lost that clipboard, I would be com-pletely lost.

When they find the right medication that doesn't have too many bad side-effects, many dys-tonia patients are satisfied to take the pills several times a day and to carry on their lives relatively normally. However, medication in the form of pills may not be suitable for many persons.

Another option is injection into an affected muscle of an agent that blocks nerve impulses as they travel from brain to muscle. Developed since 1980, the substance injected is a solution of botulinum toxin, better known to most people as a poison that grows inside a jar or can of beans that was improperly processed. For clinical use, of course, beans are not involved. The processing of botulinum toxin is meticulous, and dosages are carefully monitored so that its poisonous effects are much reduced. According to a position statement issued by the American Academy of Neurology in 1989, botulinum toxin type A (called "BOTOX" by the manufacturer) is safe and effective for several neurological applications, including certain types of dystonia.

Steve finally tried these injections after several years of treatment failure and even agonizing side-effects from other medications.

Describe your botulinum-toxin injections.

I made an appointment with Dr. Jankovic [chief neurologist at the Movement Disorders Clinic, Baylor College of Medicine, Houston TX]. I had heard about BOTOX. So we drove to Houston, I got injected, and the position I was in ... like that [moves head and neck to turned position]. They injected this muscle—lower sterno-cleido-mastoid—and that shrunk, shrunk back in, and then I was left just crooked but not that [returns head to former, nearly normal position]. At the time of BOTOX treatment Dr. Jankovic was up-front with me. He did EMG examinations and he said he felt he could help me somewhat in this front area and relieve some of the abnormal posture, but he said, "Your pain source is in the para-spinal muscle. The

61

contractions are taking place ... we only go in three and a half inches," is what he said, "with the probes to measure muscle activity." He said, "You're registering a level five on a zero-to-five scale of muscle contraction at the three-and-a-half-inch level." He said, "I don't think BOTOX will ever help your pain," and he was up front with me. But he said he could help some of the abnormal posturing by injecting this muscle, which I have had injected over the years several times. That's been helpful.

I don't see that your muscle is abnormal now.

No, this muscle's fine. This muscle's basically fine.

It looks as though it's relaxed.

It's relaxed. The BOTOX has been supremely helpful.

———

Botulinum toxin (type A), when it is helpful, usually provides relief for three or four months. After that, the effect wears off, and the muscle typically returns to its previous state of tension or spasm. But temporary relief is only part of the caution dystonia patients must have. They also need to know that some muscles are smaller and easier to reach than others; that limitation severely affects the usefulness of botulinum toxin (type A) for many patients. It's the smaller muscles around the eyes and in other parts of the face, the vocal cords, and certain muscles in the neck that are easiest to reach and are most likely to respond favorably.

Joe, a New-York-City businessman, has cervical dystonia. He asked me to sit to his left as we talked so that he could favor that side. His head turns only slightly away from normal now, but that's because he continues to get BOTOX shots.

Weren't you among the first people in the United States to get botulinum-toxin injections?

It wasn't until '87 when I joined an early experimental group that was getting BOTOX shots that I really saw any form of medication to have benefit. Also, before I get into that, I did physical therapy as well. I had a wonderful physical therapist work on my neck, turning it and massaging it gently in the hopes that that would free up these poorly functioning muscles. That made me feel good for the moment but didn't help at all. So when I had my first series of BOTOX I didn't feel any benefit at all. Went back again and found it to be very beneficial. And at first I thought I was in the control group that had just saline in the neck and not the BOTOX. I learned later I had had the injections the first time, and the fact it had no benefit was just the luck of the draw, and the second time it did and I've been helped by BOTOX ever since.

So that's, I guess, almost seven years that I've been using it but not a lot. I'm fortunate that my case is not extreme. To me, any change is extreme but it's not the serious types of cases that I have seen that are far worse even than just torticollis. And so I limit the amount of BOTOX I get in any year 'cause I don't want to ever develop the antibodies. I always want BOTOX to be there for me, so I take it probably less than I should. I think it's been fourteen months since my last series. I'm getting ready to have it again. I just always want that treatment and I don't ever want to have antibodies because it certainly is a help to me. I'm a big devotee of the product because it works.

Do you determine when you need a new set of shots according to how severe the turning is becoming again?

Well, yes, it's how much strain I feel in the neck and actually it's beginning to be also told by the feelings I get in my fingers—my fingers start getting numb and that's all because of disk involvement—that the head turns more and more, which compresses the spinal column, and that then starts closing off the nerve endings and that's how I begin to tell myself, "You're letting it go too long." I get the shots. It straightens the neck out, relieves the pressure from the disks, and then I'm better till the next time. And I learned that actually when I was going to have surgery, three and a half years ago, because of the disks. I was having numbness in the fingers, and I went to an orthopedic surgeon, who gave me the straight orthopedic route: I had the MRIs, I had the CT scans, I had all of the treatments to prove that I had disk problems, which I do. And before I was going to have surgery, I went to Columbia [University] and had shots. And just the fact of the head being twisted and turned and being alleviated by the BOTOX took the head back straight, took the pressure off the spinal column, and I didn't need surgery. So now I'm beginning to understand that, when I go too long and the head starts to turn a little bit too much, it puts pressure on the spinal column and so I have to have the shots again. And that's what I'm starting to feel now. All these wonderful things you learn about your own body that you didn't know before!

———————

Joe's reference to antibodies is another of the concerns facing a patient who wants to try botulinum toxin (type A). Some scientific evidence has accumulated to suggest that the body may, indeed, develop an immunological response to the botulinum toxin, rendering any further use inadvisable. Since there are other types of the toxin besides type A, however, they may prove useful—after further testing—to patients who have become immune to type A.

The most drastic treatment for dystonia is surgery—drastic because of its extreme invasiveness and its irreversibility. One has to comprehend the state of mind of the dystonia patient who would contemplate undergoing such surgery. Marjorie said that her decision grew out of a feeling of near desperation.

What was your state of mind at the time you decided to let a surgeon work on your neck muscles?

I was living in San Diego, so I kept calling hospitals, as I always did. I called them all in Seattle and didn't get any response, but wherever I would go I would call the hospitals to see if there was anything new developing. She said, "Oh, there's been a breakthrough." This was Neurology at Scripps Hospital. "Oh, my God," I thought and made an appointment immediately to see the doctor. He was telling me that he had several patients and that he had performed surgery [selective resection and denervation] on eleven patients, and he gave me their names so I could contact them and decide what to do. I came back to Seattle. I was very excited. I cried. I did everything. I thought, "Oh, this is so exciting. This will end everything and I'll be just perfect again and can do everything again." I returned to California and had the surgery. They had someone check me over and do the tests to find out what muscles were involved. They told me all about what would happen. He was going to cut off nerves in my neck that were causing my head to pull to one side and then the muscle. When that muscle was gone, then the head couldn't pull to one side. Anything just to relieve a person from all this constant pain.

What did the surgeon say about risks?

He said that your head could be weaker. It didn't make any difference. I didn't care. You were so tired of trying to disguise this. You were so tired of holding your head up. You were just so tired of everything. Nothing would have been bad at that point. I couldn't work any more. I couldn't do any of the things I wanted to do.

I stayed down there for six weeks for physical therapy. They said the physical therapy was the most important thing to straighten everything out. And if you didn't do that, you might as well not have the surgery. They have special exercises for that, and you're supposed to do them two or three times a day after the surgery. For example, you lay down on the bed, you lift your head up, and then you turn it to the sides. You dip your head. You do them slowly, like stretching. You start with five of a particular exercise, and you gradually go up to how many you can do. You have weights that you lift—smaller ones for your arms because the arms are so weak. My arms are always weak because there's still pain that comes down to the elbows each day. It didn't get rid of this. I don't know if this is just part of the disease or if this is from the arthritis that has set in or what. But I think it's just from so long that I had the disease—the pulling for so many years. This is just part of the dystonia. I don't think you ever get rid of the disease. I got rid of the spasms. I don't know if my head shakes very much. Do I have a little tremor? It's still better than having the spasms.

I still suffer a lot of pain and I've chosen not to take medications anymore. I've just chosen for my body to take over. The doctor is thinking of discontinuing the surgery because it hasn't helped that many people. You have to have determination in order for it to be successful. I wanted it so desperately.

———

Another surgical technique involves destroying tissue in the basal-ganglia region of the brain. Since that is the portion of the brain believed to be most involved in transmitting nerve impulses that activate muscle movement, the hope is to reduce the excessive number of impulses at the source.

This contrasts with botulinum toxin that works at the site of the affected muscle.

Adele, who spends most of her waking hours in a wheelchair because she can't walk, recalled her brain surgeries performed by Dr. Irving S. Cooper, a pioneering neurosurgeon, now deceased, in New York City. He developed the technique of cryosurgery: freezing and therefore destroying selected brain tissue in order to reduce or eliminate the dystonia symptoms. Adele was one of his many dystonia patients in 1972, when she was seven years old.

What led to your having brain surgery?

We went to many doctors, and I was lucky that we found Dr. Cooper in St. Barnabas in the Bronx and he diagnosed me. And he operated on me. I had cryosurgery where they freeze a little part of the brain.

The thalamus? [the thalamus is one of the structures that comprise the basal ganglia]

Yes. And after some months of therapy I was fine. I was walking and back to my old self. And about a year or a year and a half went by and my left hip started to pull, and I also had problems straightening my leg out at the knee, so we went back to the doctor and he did three more surgeries, and none of them helped. And on the last one he hit my speech center.

I was warned about that too when I was talking with a neurologist about that surgery.

Uh-huh. So I mean you're awake during the ... telling you to talk and I couldn't talk so they ended it right there. And that was my last brain surgery. I said, "You're not touching me anymore." That was the third time they tried to help me and I said, "You're not going into my head anymore."

Tell me a little more about your feelings about having that kind of surgery. Were you apprehensive—quite apprehensive—in the first place?

Well, I was young. I was like seven years old.

Your parents were saying you should?

They never told me what to do. Everything was always left up to me, but I wanted to make my parents happy. And I thought that it might work so I did it. Yeah.

But the fourth time you were old enough to say, "I'm not going to please my parents. I'm going to please me. No more."?

No more.

———

Hazel also underwent Dr. Cooper's surgery but several years previous to Adele and with happier results.

How old were you when you had brain surgery?

I was thirteen. I had ... February 2 I had a left-side thalamotomy because at that time there were no drugs at all. The drugs were vitamins—vitamin E, vitamin B—there were no drugs that could be of any value.

And your symptoms were progressing so rapidly that you really thought you had no choice?

I had no choice. I was crawling on the floor. I couldn't walk then. I walked backwards. I could not walk forwards. I was really relieved to have a wheelchair because it was an effort. The wheelchair wasn't allowed in school because this was 1960—no rights or anything.

By that time was it affecting all parts of your body—midsection too?

Yeah. I was bent over and backwards, like a question mark. Somebody wrote an article on me—"Little Miss Question Mark." I was more like all the way down to the floor. I couldn't bend the leg forward. It was an impossibility. There was no medication. Everyone told me there was nothing that could be done.

How much pain at that point?

I don't believe ... I don't remember. So I don't know if I had no pain or if I just don't remember.

You don't remember your muscles feeling tight and hard?

I think I was too concerned with being, you know, different and an adolescent. I can't remember the pain. I've looked at photos of myself during those years, and I don't look happy at all—just sadder and sadder.

At age thirteen that would be a big concern.

I can't remember ... so many horrible notions at that time—going to school and crawling upstairs, downstairs, being rejected, going to a hotel for a summer vacation and being asked to leave ... everything has happened. I don't know. I don't remember the pain. Maybe it was just too intense. Everything was heightened, though, obviously. What I do remember is that day on the operating table, I suddenly felt this rush of relief. Sudden relaxation when they told me. I was in miserable pain because they put your head in clamps and it hurts terribly. The pneumo-encephalogram at that time hurt terribly, and then I suddenly felt this relief, and I knew that I'd be able to use my right arm and my right leg somewhat better. I can remember that.

Were they stimulating or touching different parts of the thalamus and then asking you...?

Yeah, I guess they were. They were trying to see how big a lesion to make, and when they hit the right spot, I knew it. I was awake and I was talking and I said, "It feels better." And probably told them some other nonsense, but I do remember that vividly. Obviously there must have been a lot of tension, but I can remember the moment of release, which is probably good. So while I was screaming about other things, I had this release.

Then three months later Dr. Cooper asked my permission to operate again, and my parents and I agreed to go ahead in May, 1962. Both sides were affected terribly. I couldn't write very well. I did have a typewriter, which I only recently got rid of because I bought a new one. I was just attached to it. But I still couldn't walk very well. I was undergoing a lot of physical therapy—three times a week. I literally did not know how to put one foot in front of the other. I had to be taught. I went to the top place. I went to Rush Institute. I lived in New York. It was easy to go to the best place. I thought, well, if I could get a little better, like my friend Joan [who had also been Dr. Cooper's surgical patient], then maybe I wouldn't need this wheelchair because in school I couldn't use the wheelchair. They wouldn't allow it because of liability, so it was still a struggle. My classmates were very helpful to me but I couldn't easily get around. The left side was still getting worse. I knew that. It wasn't going to get better on its own, so I said, "Why not?" The second surgery was a right-side thalamotomy. It worked very well. And for seven years I was just about normal.

Hazel is in middle age now, working regularly at a rigorous job in the mental-health field. Some of her dystonia symptoms have recurred, but they are not nearly as severe as they were during her adolescence. She walks independently, talks fluently though with a slight impediment, and maintains an extremely positive attitude.

Chapter 5

Maintaining a Satisfactory Quality of Life

Dystonia can be a very heavy burden—affecting nearly every aspect of one's daily life, from brushing one's teeth to maintaining a marriage and earning a living. The effects may seem minor, at least to an observer, when the muscle tension is not crippling, though even the non-crippling forms of dystonia take a psychological toll, through embarrassment and a tendency to withdraw from social situations. For those whose bodies are twisted and beset by constant pain, the effects—again to an observer—may seem catastrophic.

Most of the people I interviewed admitted to having had some very dark times: periods when they felt self-pity, anger, and even considered the possibility of suicide. But with help from friends and family or simply through their own gritty determination not to be defeated, they have found something positive about their situations and have resolved to maintain, if not a fully satisfactory quality of life, at least a tolerable one.

Joseph is in his late twenties, seriously affected by generalized dystonia. His speech was painfully slow and difficult to understand; each sentence took minutes, not seconds, to utter, and his mother had to "translate" so that I could fully understand. His arms moved uncontrollably. When he attempted to walk, he lurched from chair to wall to table, trying to maintain his balance and to move his legs rhythmically. Despite these obvious limitations, though, he offered surprising information about what he **can** do.

Are the symptoms stable now?

It stopped progressing about seven or eight years ago.

Could you describe what you are able to do now?

I can still ride a bike. I can still play pool. I don't feel like I have been stopped from doing things that other people can do.

Do you drive a car?

Uh-huh.

You live alone?

Right.

You do your own cooking?

Yes. I can use a microwave. I maintain my household. I vacuum.

You mentioned that you ride a bicycle and play pool. That requires certain kinds of coordination that maybe would be surprising to some people. When you do certain kinds of movement, do some of your dystonia symptoms lessen or disappear? For instance, some people who have dystonia can't walk very well, but they can run.

Right. I can run better than I can walk.

Describe playing pool. Your arms need to be in fine adjustment, right?

Yeah, but I've been playing since I was like five.

Tell me how you handle the coordination that pool requires.

It's a mystery.

You use a computer, right? Tell me about typing.

I type with one finger, but I have become quite fast—about 40 words a minute.

Do you have your own computer?

Uh-huh.

I suppose you come out with very few mistakes because they're easy to fix.

Right.

Do you notice that when you first wake up after sleeping the symptoms are less?

Uh-huh. I can walk, talk, and everything is just fine.

For how long?

About one hour.

After about an hour, do the symptoms seem the same every day or do they vary from day to day?

They vary from hour to hour.

Getting worse as the day goes along?

Sometimes. I take a nap about half way through to reenergize my body.

When you wake up from the nap, is it like it was when you woke up in the morning?

Right.

Has it affected your eyes at all?

No.

You're able to read easily?

Uh-huh.

Let's talk about some of the reactions that you've had to this. I'm sure that after 18 years with dystonia you can remember a whole range of reactions. What were some of the first reactions when you were 13?

Most of my closest friends were confused. But then after I started using marijuana, they thought that was what was causing it.

How did you react then? Were you embarrassed?

Actually I was quite proud of this reputation that I had.

Do you think you would have been proud if you were older? Was it because you were a rebellious teenager?

Yes.

What was the next reaction you can remember having?

Severe depression.

At 16? 17?

17.

Did that continue for months, years?

That would come and go off and on till I was about 22.

Was one of the reasons for feeling more depressed that the symptoms were getting more severe?

That was one reason. I had become more involved with other recreational drugs was the other reason.

You saw a connection between using the drugs and the depression?

Yes.

I don't know how much you want to say about this, but do you think you were somehow inclined to use more drugs to cover up the symptoms, or was it just to get yourself feeling better in the head?

It was an addiction. What had once been fun had become out of control.

What can you say now about having dystonia and wanting to use drugs? Certainly you weren't the only one at the time who was experimenting with drugs. Do you think you were more likely to do that because of the dystonia?

I think it was for acceptance.

Was the dystonia making you feel less accepted?

Right.

I suppose during that period it was hard for you to sort out whether people were reacting to you because of the drugs or reacting to you because of the dystonia. They probably got kind of mixed up. What were some of the reactions you recall from close friends and family?

Lots of pity.

They would say, "Oh, I feel so sorry for you"?

They wouldn't come out and say it but I could sense it. Plus, my mother and father became obsessed with me. Friendships began to drop off because they couldn't understand what was going on.

And neither could you?

Right.

Was that adding to your depression?
Most definitely.

How did teachers react to you? You had difficulty, I suppose, doing assignments.
Right.

Did they kind of accept your failure? Maybe sidestepping confronting you about doing the work?
Well, I was such a troublemaker that I think they just kind of pushed me aside.

Did anyone tell you you needed to be in a special-education class?
In high school, I was.

What happened there? Were the teachers different there?
No.

Did you try to get out of doing work?
As much as possible.

When you think about the positive and the negative aspects of having dystonia, what has been positive about it? Have you felt hope or encouragement in any form? Have you been aware of what you could do more than you might have if you hadn't had the disability? A lot of us take for granted doing things that you can't do or can't do successfully. But maybe you're more aware of what you can do.
If it hadn't been for having this, I don't think I would be as intellectual. I'd probably be like my uncles.

When people wake up in the morning, they have a general feeling about facing the day— looking forward to doing interesting things, meet-

ing interesting people. Some people wake up and think, "Oh, God, I don't want to get out of bed." How is it for you usually?

Now I look forward to each day because now I have goals. I have an active social life.

And you can do many of the things that you enjoy doing, apparently. Do you want to tell me what some of your goals are, if they aren't too personal?

I would like to write for a national fashion publication someday. Right now, I'm writing for a weekly newspaper.

So writing is pretty high on your list of goals?

Uh-huh. I'd like to make lots of money.

Why do you need—or want—lots of money? That probably seems like a silly question to you.

I don't settle for second best that often, if at all possible. I like to have the best clothes. I like to have the nicest apartment, etcetera, etcetera.

Do you feel that you need to make up for things that you missed out on or weren't able to do when you were younger? So this would be one way of getting what you think you deserve?

I feel like after my ten years of drug addiction and alcoholism, I missed out on a lot of stuff I could have done.

Do you have a pet?

Yes. A cat.

Tell me about your feelings about the cat.

Well, Warhol is my best friend.

How old is he?

Two years.

Is he your first pet?

He's my first pet of my own.

What does he do for you that people don't—or can't?

He makes me laugh. He's always there. And he's always glad to see me.

I suppose there are times when you feel discouraged.

Not so much nowadays.

Is that because you've got yourself on a more even keel emotionally?

I think so.

You're stressing the things you can do and the goals. So that balances out any reasons for being discouraged?

Right.

David greeted me from a prone position on the floor of his apartment, saying, "You'll have to excuse me, but I feel most comfortable when I'm at home just crawling around on the floor." His apology lacked all self-consciousness. I joined him on the floor so we could talk eye-to-eye. Lying on his stomach and bracing himself with powerful arms, he spoke clearly and with sustained vigor, though his legs would obey few of his commands to move in a desired way. He made it clear that his condition would be much worse—even less control over movement—if it were not for his medications of both prescription drugs and BOTOX injections.

David is in his early thirties and has had generalized dystonia since he was about seven years old. He recalled his early realization that for him, his intellect—because dystonia has no effect on anyone's intellectual functioning—might make up for whatever physical limitations he had.

Were you going to school when your dystonia symptoms appeared?

I was going to school which ... the Elysee Francais, which is a French school. My mother wanted me to learn French very much. She was French. My mother was summoned, almost, to the school at one point, when I was something like nine—before I went into a wheelchair—and she saw in the principal that he was about to say, "Well, your child should no longer be in this school." My mother saw that and before he was able to spit out those words, she said, "Well, I have to take my son out of this school." I was always very proud of the fact that she saw what was coming and instead of him making the move, she made the move.

I studied for approximately two years using home schooling, and my mother, who was a staff member at the United Nations, got an interview for me at the United Nations International School. That was a school that was composed ... that represented basically the United Nations. Being different—quote, unquote—meant absolutely nothing in that school. That was not the reason my mother thought of it. That was not the reason that anyone thought that that would be the best school, but, upon reflection, when I was 20 or 25 or whatever age I was, I thought back. I said, "Oh, that's why I was accepted so readily in that school by the other students: 'Oh, this is just another different person—slightly different person—who has a different background, who has different attributes, who has a slightly different look, but who is as intelligent as we are." The mental faculties are not affected. "So, you know, we'll copy his homework if it's good, and we'll let him copy our homework if he hasn't done something," etcetera.

And since writing has been very difficult if not impossible since the age of maybe 11 or 12, so I developed a very good memory. I went through the United Nations International School, which goes up to high school. I graduated from that with honors, etcetera, etcetera. I went to Columbia University, which I finished in 3 years. I took a lot of classes during the summer, and I also got some advanced placement because I had completed some courses which were really college-level courses in high school. And then NYU [New York University] School of Law from 1982 to 1985.

So how old are you now?

I just turned 32 on April 4.

So it's 25 years ...

I just turned 32, and, yeah, there's still some hair left.

You've had obviously quite a lot of time to think this over and draw some inferences about having dystonia. I'd be interested in your observations on some of the psychological effects.

Since it was an early onset ... I have thought about it a bit, especially after my mother passed away. For some reason I did think about it. I believe, since the dystonia was an early onset—around the age of seven or eight—that I was not deprived—quote, unquote—of being able to do something—not the same as in your case, for example.

Something that you had already been doing but suddenly had to stop doing?

Yes. I had not driven a car. I had not done a lot of things which adults are able, legally, to do. It was not that much of a psychological impact on me, and the students at the United Nations School made me feel ... I did not have the ostracized feeling at all. It was not "Oh, this ... let's leave him in the corner" type of thing. I did not have that feeling at all. In fact, the principal at the school said, "You would be surprised but your being here is an incredible asset for the school and for other students. Maybe you might not realize it but they are seeing a person who is in a wheelchair, who is doing the exact same thing that they are doing, who is helping them with their homework when they need help with their homework," etcetera, etcetera, "doing what 13-, 14-, 15-year-old kids do normally, and," he said, "that's having a profound impact on the way they will grow up and the way they will look at the world thirty years from now or even less."

That must have been crucial, really, to find out what self-esteem can consist of.

I don't know if I absorbed that sentence completely when it was told to me ...

Not then.

Not then, but I remembered it now, yeah. But to go back, when I graduated from law school in 1985, that's when I hit the real world.

Tell me, just briefly, why did you decide to do law school?

Uhhh ... one of my father's favorite sentences always was "Brains over brawn." And I very much liked the analytical way of thinking in law school. I think, in fact, from high school, Columbia University was just a stop-off point. I knew in high school that I wanted to go to law school. I didn't know which one, but I knew I wanted to go to law school.

When you did enter law school, was it with the idea that you might then practice law in some form?

Yes, it was.

And have you done that?

That's when I was saying ... in 1985 that's when I hit the real world. I think I applied to ... for probably about 250 different positions—in different corporations, for the federal government, for the state government, city. It didn't matter, whatever level. And the letters would always read, "You have a very good resume, but ..." And I sort of got used to that: "You have a very good resume, but..."

"But" being followed by something that's clearly discriminatory?

No, you have to remember that I was being declined by lawyers, and lawyers on paper will never put down ...

Isn't that what it amounted to, though?
Of course.

Were you telling them, or did they know before they considered you that your body is as it is?

Yes, I always told them. I always include ... I don't include that on my resume, but what I do include on a covering letter, "If travel is required..." I've basically travelled around the world for very extended periods of time, and it hasn't been a problem.

Well, what would you say, then, is the real reason that they don't want to hire you in their firms?

I believe what they are most concerned about is the interface between me and the public at large.

Well, there must be all kinds of attorney positions that don't involve a lot of that—where they deal with a telephone.

Exactly. If there was a back room ... at that time there weren't ... everyone was really out front. If you wanted to be a clerk or a researcher for someone, I probably could apply for that and I would be able to do that.

Do you still want to?

That's the question. I don't. I tried to pass the bar exam six different times, and the bar exam is given on Tuesday and Wednesday every single time, and I would try to gain as much strength as I could. I would do well on Tuesday, poor on Wednesday. I would look at the results and I would say, "Oh, I have to put more energies into Wednesday." So then I would do ... I would fail because

I've had very low scores on Tuesday and very good scores on Wednesday.

The people who give the bar exam are not about to accommodate anybody with any kind of special need, huh?

This was before the Americans with Disabilities Act. Several times I wrote letters to their executive director, saying basically, "Look, for the bar exam why don't you give it to me on Tuesday? On Wednesday, I'll pay for the hotel room, I'll pay for the security guard, you can rip out the phone if you want. You can sequester me in that sense. What I need is a day of downtime, a day where I can just lie down, do nothing, or just watch television. I'm not interested in cheating on the test. I'm just interested in being able to take examinations on the same par as other students." The answer was always "No. No, we can't do that. Security might be breached," etcetera, etcetera.

How about a suit that would help a few other people too?

Yeah. Well, it was before the Americans with Disabilities Act.

But it's not too late if it became a cause.

Yeah, if it became a cause. I could do it now, probably, and I could use the Americans with Disabilities Act as a club almost, for lack of a better word, but when you take the bar exam or a lot of other exams, you have to have, again for lack of a better word, the fire in the belly. You really have to be able to wake up at 8:00 or 7:30 or whatever it is, drink a cup of coffee, eat something for breakfast, and then study for four or five hours, then stop, eat lunch in about a half an hour, then start again and study for another six hours. Basically, television is ... OK, you catch the nightly news and that's it. And everything else is devoted to studying, and this basically lasts for two to four weeks, and it takes a lot out of you—studying for the exam, besides just taking it. Studying for the exam really takes a lot out of you. I don't know ... in fact, I do know that right now, I don't have the incentive, nor do I really want to put myself through that. Everyone is telling me or a lot of people have told me, "Do it," etcetera, etcetera, but they're not the ones that are going to do the studying. I'm the one who has to do the studying, and you basically have to turn your life over to books for two to four weeks.

———

During my two-hour conversation with David, we veered to many subjects beyond dystonia. I finally felt comfortable in asking him about the spiritual side of his life: whether he thought his physical condition had somehow brought him to a higher spirituality. He began by citing the Koran, Robert Oppenheimer, Isaac Newton, and Einstein, all of whom he considered shaping influences of his spirituality.

Has your almost-lifelong dystonia actually strengthened you emotionally or spiritually?

I am agnostic in not believing in a particular religion but I'm not atheistic. I do believe that there's some higher power out there that either was involved in forming the universe or is controlling things somehow, and I don't know how. I don't know why that's happening. It might be proven or disproven or never explored, but those ... it has been explored ... but those are things which I always keep ... that's something I always keep in the back of my mind. I always keep the nay-saying atti-tude in the back of my mind.

Would it be fair to say, then, as a result of that, that you are able to think of your inability to walk as a trivial problem?

I don't even think of it. I don't even think of my inability to walk. Getting into my wheelchair is almost auto ... not almost automatic, is automatic.

I suppose because it has been practically your whole life.

Exactly.

So if you look around and you see others and maybe you think, "Well, if I could ... so and so ..."

No. I've passed by so many playgrounds where the kids are playing basketball or whatever, and I'll just watch through the fence and admire some of the stuff that some of the players might be doing on the playground, but my mind never wan-ders to the point of saying, "Well, dyston ... if I didn't have dystonia, then maybe I would be able to also play with these players." That thought just never crosses my mind. Again, that goes back to not being deprived of something.

Not feeling deprived of something is a state less often achieved by people whose dystonia struck in adulthood. Daniel is an example of a man whose life took an abrupt shift 20 years ago, when, after being in an automobile accident, he started having neck spasms. Now in his 50s, he spends his days in a semi-drifting state, able to perform routine tasks and to go for occasional walks. He has tried numerous drugs and has had stereotactic brain surgery in Germany. Some treatments made the symptoms worse; he has only slight hope that he will find a better treatment.

How have you found yourself reacting emotionally to all of this? Over 20 years, I'm sure there have been lots of ups and downs.

Yes, lots of ups and downs. I got very depressed.

More downs than ups?

If I may say that, I don't like to talk about it, but for the benefit of accuracy, I tried to kill myself several times in the garage, with carbon monoxide and with pills. Obviously, I wasn't very successful, but it has strained relations—is straining relations—terribly with my son also, who I couldn't pay a lot of attention to. He's 21 years old now. I couldn't do very many things with him because of my torticollis, and he holds that before me all the time.

Of course, he was an infant when you first got this, wasn't he?

One year old. In the beginning when I lost control over my functions, I had terrible anxiety attacks. I didn't even know what the anxiety attacks were until I had several of them. It's terrible.

Generalized anxiety or focused on something?

No, it was generalized. One day, I remember, I was over on Vashon Island [near Seattle] with friends of mine, and I had drunk a strong cup of coffee and I had taken a very strong sleeping pill the night before, and I walked outdoors into the sunlight and all of a sudden I had to walk in circles around. My heart beat like crazy.

Have you had any kind of psychologist's help?

Yes, I must say I had two attempts at psychoanalysis, sort of. The doctor I saw writes beautiful bills. But that didn't help.

Maybe some more limited form of psychotherapy would help.

He also suggested to my wife that I was doing this to anger her.

Well, I suppose that makes you cautious about seeing anybody else.

That's right.

What do you find gives you the greatest strength and encouragement?

If I can read a book. When I have no medication, my spasms are more severe and I cannot read a book. I lose my line all the time. I finished several books lately. When I read, the time flies by, and it's interesting.

Would you enjoy doing more things with other people?

Yes, I would like to go on hikes. I would like to work. I really would like to work.

What kind of work had you been doing?
I was service manager for Volkswagen.
Some other kind of work perhaps?
Yeah. I cannot concentrate very long.
But you concentrate on a book?
Yeah. That seems to be easy.

———————

Later in the interview, Daniel spontaneously summarized the dystonia experience for him, saying, "I don't know if I'm overstating this, but it ruined my life."

I talked to Lucy, who is physically more disabled than Daniel, in her apartment. She had left the door ajar, preferring not to bother maneuvering her battery-powered wheelchair from her living room, through a hall, to the entry door. Though she does get out of the apartment three times a week to do volunteer work, she spends most of her time by herself. Now in her mid-thirties, she is afflicted not only by cervical dystonia and spasmodic dysphonia but also by muscular dystrophy. She's not sure which is worse: the dystonic turning of her neck and the difficulty in speaking or the general weakness of many other muscles. Both conditions seem to be progressive, despite every treatment physicians can offer.

Though Lucy has a brother who lives nearby and provides help when she asks for it, she depends on a certified nursing attendant who comes to the apartment three times a week.

You have great difficulty in moving all parts of your body. What sort of help does your assistant provide?

She comes here and she helps me with personal needs, like I can't bathe, I can't shampoo myself, and I need help dressing, and then she does the physical therapy, which is the stretching exercises. She turns my neck, which I can't do. And then she massages my back. I have a curvature of the spine, which causes me to get an inflammation.

If she's here three days a week, how do you manage on the other days?

I manage ... uh ... I get up in the morning—when she's not here or even where she is here—I get up in the morning. I get dressed and then I get in my wheelchair and then I get breakfast and I go to volunteer and I get home like 3:30 or 4:00. On Mondays the lady that comes does my meal preparation, so she makes sure I have sandwiches made or casseroles in the freezer so all I have to do is throw them in the micro. Then, after I do that, I watch TV or listen to music, whatever. Then go to bed.

Is it extremely difficult for you to manage these things yourself?

Right now, I've learned some tricks. It's difficult because I go to work at 10:00 and I have to get up at 6:00. I just can't run in the bedroom and get in a pair of jeans. I have to get my breakfast. It's real hard to eat ...

How would you describe your attitude now about all of these limitations ... and opportunities?

I'm still mad.

That's probably a good thing. If you were passive about it and too accepting, that would probably slow you down a lot. Mad in the sense of a generalized anger at whoever did this to you?

Yeah, and I don't know why. No one can tell me did I do something wrong. I didn't smoke pot or something. Did I eat something wrong?

Your mind tells you that you didn't do anything wrong, doesn't it?

Well, yeah. I didn't do anything that a normal kid didn't do. Before I was sick, I was a normal kid. You know, I got into mischief but I didn't kill anyone or do anything bad.

In the times when you're not feeling quite as angry, what's your attitude?

Frustration. I get real frustrated and I get depressed. Everything that I want help in is up to me. It's hard. Not because of the MD [muscular dystrophy] so much because all that does is keep me in the chair and it makes it a little harder. I don't belong some places. More than that, the dystonia is wreaking havoc. The MD doesn't really hold me back from doing that much. When I was just in a wheelchair, that was not pleasant, but it didn't affect me. I can't read now. There's a lot of things that I might try and do, but I know they're too stressful and they're going to aggravate the dystonia. I know I'm going to be in a lot of pain. So there's a lot of daily things that I can't do because of the dystonia.

How do you do volunteer work if there are so many "daily things" you can't do because of the dystonia?

One day a week I volunteer at the Muscular Dystrophy Association office downtown.

How do you get there?

We have a wheelchair express-van system in this area for low-income handicapped. They take me there. I go there and I file billings and I collate and I stuff envelopes—clerical.

Are those things hard for you to do?

It takes me a while, but I can do 'em. I'm not as fast but it's volunteer work.

How much satisfaction do you get out of that?

A lot. Besides it's getting me out of the house. When you're at work, as I'm sure you know, you don't have time to concentrate on any depressing thoughts or pain or stuff about you. You're just doing the work. And then I get home from work and I come in the door and then, all of a sudden— I've been in pain all day—but all of a sudden I get in the door and it's just "How can I even sit up?" It's very rewarding because not only do I get out of the house, I feel I'm doing something useful. There are people paid to do this. When I'm folding literature to be mailed to people and putting it in the envelopes, that is giving the secretary time to work on the computer or do phone calls or something that they couldn't do ... so they don't have to do menial stuff that I can do and they can do stuff that I can't do.

I suspect, though, that with your knowledge and experience, there are some kinds of activities that you could do that aren't quite so menial and that would be very important—talking to people in a kind of a counseling relationship, for example. Couldn't you do that?

Yeah, I used to. That's what I did about four years ago. On Thursday and Friday I volunteer at the resource center for the handicapped.

That's your other volunteer activity. Can you tell me about that?

Well, I love that. I like that because it's a homey atmosphere. To me it's like ... you go there and it's an office but there are only like maybe twenty people. Everyone knows everyone else and I like that.

What kinds of services do they provide?

At first it was a real resource center for the handicapped: we helped people with accessible housing; we helped people get personal-care attendants—which is what I get. That's when I interviewed and I counseled people. We had counseling, we had a lot of support groups.

Do you ever hear the word "dystonia" mentioned around there?

Never. No. I met this man. I talk about it and they all know what it is and sometimes we go into detail. The weird thing is when I started taking the BOTOX injections, I didn't know whether there was going to be a direct effect, because I don't get out into public. After about two months of the injection people noticed it. I wasn't in constant pain, or if I was it wasn't that bad. They noticed that my neck was straighter. I could do more stuff without being in constant pain because when you get in pain your face kind of scrunches up, and I was always scrunched up.

You go there Thursdays and Fridays, you said. Are you there for three or four hours each time?

No. Thursday I'm there 10:00 to 4:00, and Friday I'm there 10:00 to 2:00.

What are your main activities?

Right now I'm working in the Washington State Employment Security Office. They find jobs for disabled people. Right now the resource is totally changed. It was starting out as a resource center. Now they've totally changed it so it's just a technical school. They have five classes. If someone calls for a resource, they're referred somewhere else. So there isn't anything for me to do because I can't work in classes. I'm not a teacher, so I work in the Employment Security office putting together a job list—800 numbers, people that are looking for jobs—and call a 24-hour job line and find out every job that's available, if it's wheelchair-accessible. The people in my office get them the job, and they kind of follow up to make sure they're being successful and the company is doing what they said.

Are you yourself mainly working with paper or do you have a lot of interaction with other people—the telephone or interviews or conversations?

No. Mainly paper. Mainly it's just working computer job lines and roughing in jobs and putting them in order.

As you cast your eyes over these lists of jobs and openings and so on and think about your own desires, are there some of them you wish you could take? Other jobs you'd like to have?

Well, there are some of them that look promising but I like volunteering because it's my own time. I can take a break whenever I want to if I hurt. If I want to do something, I can just say, "Well, it's too hard."

I conclude, then, that earning money is not particularly important to you. Some people define their own self-worth by whether they're able to earn money. I gather you don't do that.

I need it. I'd like to do it. I'm like everyone from month to month. I'm barely making it. But my priority right now is getting out there and for me to get transportation without too much of a hassle and being able to be there and kind of be my own boss and do what I want.

———

Lucy, despite the difficulty in controlling her head and in speaking with a determined sound, seemed to summon up all her conviction when she said these words. She'll maintain her independence and do worthwhile things as long as she is physically able.

Clara, too, requires a battery-powered vehicle to get around easily, though she can use crutches to move from the automobile she drives to her office. As I came to know about her life with generalized dystonia, I stood in amazement at what she attempts, and usually succeeds, in doing.

Her office is not far from Long Island Jewish Hospital, where I had come to interview another person. I had planned to find my own way from the hospital to her office, but she insisted on picking me up in her car. If I had previously known the full extent of her muscular disorder, I would have implored her to let me drive. As we whizzed along the parkway, though, I could see that she was not taking irresponsible chances. Driving safely and doing many other things that might seem implausible or impossible to an observer are necessary to maintain her determination that dystonia is not going to conquer her or make her a recluse.

Clara has had generalized dystonia—both legs, both arms—since she was in fourth grade. She remembers how "my handwriting started to change" and "my foot was dragging a little." The disorder progressed so that by her late 20s or early 30s, she was becoming seriously disabled. Nevertheless, she taught school—fourth grade—married, and became the mother of two children. Despite treatments that helped control her muscular spasms, "They wouldn't let me teach anymore," she said with some resentment. And she had discovered that one daughter, too, had generalized dystonia in a form that has proven worse and more difficult to treat than

Clara's. That daughter is now 33 years old, living independently, and doing some work to earn money, though she is cruelly disabled despite all efforts at treatment.

Coping with disability has become Clara's specialty.

You appear to be a textbook example of how to do it.

I always was able to manage things, and I still ... I drive my daughter to the hospital for her treatments ... that's close to a 3-hour drive ... I'm able to help with the chairs. Physically, I can do a lot. There are other problems caused by the dystonia. There is loss of control ... unpleasant areas in a marriage and I don't know ... it's difficult to say ... I mean ... what has caused what. No one knows why I have difficulty with bladder and bowels. There still is no diagnosis that it's caused by ... although my daughter ... she went to college and because she needed to be catheterized ... the school accepts handicapped people, but they wouldn't catheterize. So I had three shifts of nurses come to her dorm to catheterize her. It became crazy. One couldn't come and I was going back and forth to Farmingdale [town on Long Island], to work, and to the emergency room. We just had to take her out. But it does seem, even though there is no diagnosis, that it is due to dystonia. Whenever she has a particularly rough time, she has to be catheterized. I have the opposite problem, but it's hard to say what has had its toll and what is caused by what.

As we know, every voluntary muscle in the body can be affected.

Right. So it does affect your life. My husband says, "Smile." I can't always smile. What I am great at doing ... I don't know many adults who do it ... are puzzles.

Jigsaw?

Jigsaw. I do one and I do a different one and I get totally absorbed. Nothing matters in time. Computers too absorb me. I love to work with computers. Those two things, and they're basically solitary things, but I can get absorbed.

There's also the possibility of making everything fit together and making things work in an orderly, predictable way. I should think that would be very attractive to you.

Again, it's very unusual. I have it on the kitchen table. I'm looking. "What is that piece there?" My husband says, "Could you please look at me?" ... I have ways. I love to work in my garden. I do have a green thumb. There are plants that I'm so tired of ... I can't make them die. I guess I have feelings about having to take care of my daughter so much and having to spend time in the hospital with her. My younger daughter really didn't have as much caring as she should have. She had asthma ... she has asthma ... and I didn't respond because anything short of brain surgery [undergone several years ago by her dystonic daughter] was trivial, and my husband tried to ... I mean I would take her to the hospital and do the right things but without being tuned in to what she was feeling. So those are, looking back, sad ... hard to look back on. I try to now. I try and be more where she is emotionally. She and her husband said my makeup was like a death mask. They took me to the store and bought me makeup, and I thought, "Gee, I'll look like an Indian." I sat them both down and I said, "I know you love me very much, but my makeup, no matter how I look, is what I want to do."

It was my psychiatrist who helped me deal with this. I didn't want to get angry at them so I just held it all in and did whatever they said. Then I thought, "There are ways of me talking to them kindly, saying 'I know you love me. I know you care about me.'" In that way, it helps. I am usually either a black or white person: either I'm for it ... my younger daughter, when she comes back, said, "Mom, you used to yell at people when they're parked in handicapped parking ... give them what-for." Last time I didn't. I said, "Mary, I'm tired, I'm just tired of yelling at people." I really think I do know what's important.

My sister and I lead very different lives, and I really think I have a better perspective on what's important, what really counts. I think that's one of the reasons I like working here [in a government office that provides services for handicapped people]. It's because I can ... I have a lot of energy ... all the medication I'm taking ... I don't get tired. I have an energy, and I try to energize the clients, make them get their pilot light lit, get them moving, get them doing it. In that way I can sort of get them doing ... not to obsess about it. I made so many mistakes in my life. So you do one thing and it's wrong, you do something else. In that way, I think this is a good outlet for me.

Sounds like the ideal one.

It is ideal. I think every client wishes ... but people in the hospital don't want them to know that I was once a client and I made it, so to speak. And for some reason they don't want me to share that. They're afraid that clients might feel that I wasn't competent ... I'm not sure. It doesn't really make much sense to me. I guess the one thing I have found when I speak to people who are physically handicapped is sometimes they've made it. So I try and understand what they're dealing with and walk even with small steps but not being afraid to try.

You sound like the textbook for how to cope with any kind of difficulty, and you say it in a way that's very comprehensible and very personal.

It works for me. It doesn't work for everyone.

And you're not giving out prescriptions.

No. I say that when I get uptight or nervous or maybe depressed, I go and dig in my garden. That really ... I mean I love digging in the garden, coming in with wet hands. I scrub my deck and I put flowers out. My mother comes up every June and I get the whole place ready for her—the plants and the deck. So I keep myself busy, occupied. Maybe what you said gives me a clue as to having control over the puzzle, making it all fit, making it come out whole, staying with it so I can make it right.

Chapter 6

Talking With a Neurologist

Since primary-care physicians often do not recognize symptoms of dystonia, people with dystonia symptoms who eventually discover what they have usually learn from a neurologist—a physician who specializes in disorders of the nervous system. It has now been clearly established that dystonia is not a muscular problem, although the symptoms show up in any of the muscles that control voluntary movement. It is not a problem centered in the mind—the conscious, reasoning, and emotional processes. Dystonia is, instead, a problem in the brain, which controls the central nervous system.

Because of their need to know a great deal about brain structure and functions, neurologists are therefore most likely to be up to date on relevant research, diagnosis, and treatment. During the past few years, when much new information about dystonia has been developed, many neurologists have expanded their knowledge of this still-mysterious disease and are able to talk about it with considerable clarity and accuracy.

Joseph Tsui (pronounced CHOY) is one such neurologist, who for the past 15 or more years has focused his practice and research on dystonia. A member of the staff at the Movement Disorders Centre, University of British Columbia, he has seen hundreds of patients with dystonia from Canada and the United States. He examined and videotaped my dystonic arm and hand movements in the mid-1980s and pronounced my condition untreatable by any techniques then available.

Dr. Tsui is an easy man to talk with and a fountain of information that he makes easily understandable to his patients. Here, in Dr. Tsui's own words, are answers to questions that almost any dystonia patient—or his or her family member—might wish to ask.

O.K. You say I have dystonia. What caused it? Did I inherit it? Or was it caused by some injury or bacteria?

Unfortunately we still don't know what causes dystonia. Now there are many kinds of dystonia. At least, it can be classified into the group that has the onset in young children—generalized dystonia, hereditary, particularly in Ashkenazi Jews. The marker for a gene has already been isolated in the past few years. But how does the gene lead to dystonia? We still don't know. Particularly difficult to explain is how people get focal dystonia. That is, how do they get dystonia in only one part of the body—in an adult who does not seem to have any family history of similar problems? This is the thing that we still don't know.

Is that why so many doctors have seemed to know so little about dystonia and what to do about it?

Because the doctors couldn't do anything about dystonia, they tended to ignore it years ago. And when they saw a patient with dystonia, they may not even have made a diagnosis, and even if they made a diagnosis they just said, "You have dystonia but I can't do anything about it." Patients got disappointed and therefore this condition has been left in the air for a long time.

How common is dystonia? I ask that because most doctors don't recognize it, and most people I talk to have never heard the word. They think I'm talking about that eastern European country named Estonia.

For cervical [he pronounces it *ser VI kull*] dystonia the prevalence is 8.9 per hundred thousand, or 89 per million. Now this is the figure that has frequently been quoted, and this only comes from one publication by Dr. J. Nutt, who is now in Oregon but did the study on patients in Rochester NY. This is a very old set of figures. I must say that it is probably a gross underestimate. The peak age is 40 to 49 years and it is slightly more common in females than in males—1.7 to 1.

The number of patients that we have seen in our centre up to 1992 was 622—213 from the greater Vancouver area in British Columbia, our local area. I must say with some pride that we have actually seen probably all the patients who require treatment in our local area because the awareness of dystonia is so good in our community now. It used to take seven years for patients to walk around and get the correct diagnosis when we first started the program. This has already been shortened to within a year in our community in British Columbia for the past two years.

According to the statistics, the greater Vancouver area probably has a population of about 1.5 million. According to that, it would give us a figure of 14.2 per hundred thousand, compared with the old figure of 8.9. This is a lot more—probably over 50% more. This is just for cervical dystonia, not to mention other forms of dystonia—generalized dystonia, writer's cramp, etc.

But writer's cramp is a little bit more difficult to study epidemiologically because most patients do not have very disabling symptoms, and some of them can change to the other hand to write so they may not be handicapped at all. To have an accurate figure it may actually mean a very complicated door-to-door survey or questionnaire.

Exactly how do you diagnose a patient who comes in with symptoms that might indicate dystonia?

When we see a patient coming in with a twisted neck, with a detailed history one can frequently make a diagnosis clinically. It is really a diagnosis clinically because there is no test, no lab test or any investigations to confirm it. But obviously we need to exclude a list of secondary causes. The important category is to think about whether there are any bony abnormalities in the site because sometimes it may not be surprising to take an X-ray of the neck, and it may show some congenital abnormality like a missing block on one side of the vertebra. The head is tilted to one side, but a history usually dates back much longer. Also traumatic injury: fractures of the spine compress it asymmetrically so the head is twisted. So it's always worthwhile just taking a plain X-ray of the neck. It's non-invasive and not very expensive. Sometimes it may produce some striking abnormality.

Ocular abnormality is very rare. Some patients can have some damage to the nerve going to the muscles in the eye; therefore, the eyes are looking in different directions, but they can compensate for this double vision. If the eyes are crossed, they look into one image and that is split into two. That's called double vision. They can compensate for it by tilting the head and the vision becomes one again, but this is rather rare.

Inner-ear problems: when they have inner-ear damage they need to tilt the head to a position so they do not stimulate the inner ear. Once they put the head in a different position it may produce the sensation of vertigo, or spinning around, like motion sickness.

If dystonia symptoms originate because of a problem in the brain, have you neurologists studied the brain enough to know what's really going on there?

Attempts have been done. This is a condition of motor control and therefore lots of programs in motor control are involved with that. There have been recent publications on the use of PET scans— PET meaning positron emission tomography—in writer's cramp, for example. When you activate certain movements, then certain areas of the brain can light up. They pick up some very subtle abnormalities—that is, a little deviation compared with the normal. But all these are so embryonic in their development that they are so difficult to interpret. We don't even have a good pattern for normal.

What we understand currently I can only put into a very simple example. The basal ganglia is likened to something like a computer—a computer chip. To simplify it, it seems to contain all the complex movement patterns of the body and store them in terms of programs. These programs are stored there when we're young. You learn certain complex movements. You learn to play a piano and when you're young the basal ganglia is a very plastic structure. It accepts all sorts of programming, but once the programs are there, and as one grows older, this plasticity is lost. That is, you learn things with much more difficulty when you are getting older.

These programs are interconnected with each other, executing through the cortex so we can do several things at the same time. I can talk to you, but I can also get my hand and play around with it without even thinking about it. Then I am just pulling on a few switches. These are all activated like computer switches. But in dystonia some of these programs go wrong, particularly in focal dystonia. In writer's cramp, for example, the writing program goes wrong, but the hand is completely normal doing any other things. When you want to flip on the switch of writing, it starts going crazy. The interesting issue is that there are at least two writing programs—one using the wrist and fingers, the other by using more proximal shoulder movements. Now most patients with writer's cramp when they write have problems, but when they use chalk to write on a blackboard, they are all right. They can write perfectly well.

So all this helps us to understand that it is actually much more complex than a computer—that there are motor-programming problems within the basal ganglia, and, if something goes wrong there, the action will be abnormal. That area also governs the normal posture of different parts of the body, so if that program goes wrong and it decides that the neck should be twisted, then unfortunately the brain would have to listen to this program.

So we believe that it is probably a biochemical abnormality, but even that conclusion is standing on shaky grounds. Because right now if you believe in the connections, maybe the biochemical substance there is correct but the connections are wrong. But the theory about this biochemical imbalance is that, in some patients with dystonia, you can improve the dystonia by giving them therapeutic agents like anti-cholinergic drugs, and therefore we think that it may be a biochemical imbalance.

But unfortunately not all patients respond to the same drugs. A well-known example is that—if you know the transmitter called dopamine for Parkinson's disease—some patients respond very well to dopamine, that is, a drug that enhances dopamine. But some other patients respond to drugs that oppose dopamine, and so we are completely at a loss. We are confused. Drugs that work in totally different directions can be beneficial in one patient and vice versa in another patient, and it is only dopamine.

Then we come to talk about cholinergic substances. People have been using anti-cholinergic drugs, and there has been a report on cholinergic substances—that is again a different direction—that work well in the same kind of illness. The more convincing issue is that some patients with neck dystonia can come with a history that initially the head turns to the left and after awhile turns to the right. So we don't really know what everything means. In writer's cramp, for example, some patients will start off having problems with the right hand, then shift to the use of the left hand to write. A small proportion of these patients actually after years develop the same problem in the other hand. This also helps to support the fact that it may be a central problem rather than a more peripheral problem. The theories are not very well founded. It could be a biochemical imbalance, but I suspect that in some patients, particularly in specific problems, it may be something more subtle than a biochemical imbalance.

You've talked about neck dystonia as the most common kind. What is involved?

Neck dystonia has three components. The cardinal components are sustained or persistent abnormal posturing of the head and neck and may be superimposed on top of it by intermittent movements, or jerky movements or even tremor, and it can be associated with a lot of pain. Now these three can be combined in different proportions. Some may have pain predominantly and much less abnormal posturing, and some may have more movements than persistent, abnormal posturing. These are the three cardinal features.

As far as pain goes, it can originate from different sources. It can originate from muscle spasms around the neck, but it can also come from secondary causes: if the patient has the torticollis for a long time, it may bring about degeneration of the cervical spine, in which case it can produce pain in itself. It can also produce pain radiating down the arm, but all these are secondary causes of pain rather than directly caused by the dystonia itself.

There is another feature here which may help us to make the diagnosis of idiopathic neck dystonia, and that is what we call sensory tricks or proprioceptive tricks. This is the phenomenon which describes the fact that, although the head is persistently twisted to one side, when people touch their head or neck or face anywhere, they can bring the head back straight for a brief period of time. In some of these patients they may even maintain the correct head posture for a long time, but most of these patients can do it for a short time before the head goes back. This phenomenon is absent in all those patients who have a wry neck due to a variety of secondary causes.

Well, if you don't know what causes dystonia, or if it has more than one possible cause, how can you treat it? Or do you sometimes have to say, "You'll just have to live with it"?

Anything short of knowledge of the underlying cause we really cannot provide a cure for the condition. Symptomatic treatments for the condition with all the medications have been very unsatisfactory. Most patients get temporary relief but the side-effects are so bad that most of them would finally give up the medications, and therefore it is not good at all.

Although it is not a cure, botulinum toxin provides a very good symptomatic relief for many patients. It has provided at least some hope and also given the doctors something to do to help the patient. And that actually significantly improved the awareness of the condition. Lots of research has been done, and the funding agencies have paid more attention to funding research in dystonia.

Botulism: the first reported case was in 1897. The word comes from the Latin word for sausages—food poisoning from sausages, bad sausage.

Two types of neurotoxins have been identified initially—type A and type B neurotoxin. More and more protein types of the toxin have been found—to 1970 up to 7 types described: A, B, C, D, E, F, G (C further subdivided into 1 and 2). In 1924 the bacterium was finally given a name, *clostridium botulinum*. All neurotoxins are inactivated by boiling, and only A, B, E, F have been shown to give rise to human clinical botulism. Only type A has been a marketed drug, though type F was recently investigated and shown to be effective in patients who have grown resistant to type A; the duration of effectiveness was much shorter—weeks rather than months. Type B toxin is currently being investigated in a multi-center study.

What the toxin does in the body is to go to a junction between nerves and muscles, and it blocks the impulses between nerves and muscles. Normally what happens is that, when you want the arm to move or want to contract a certain muscle of the arm, your brain sets off an electrical impulse that is conducted by a nerve like a piece of wire right down to the junction between the nerve and the muscle. But it is not electricity that goes through to the muscle. At the end of the nerve it releases a chemical, and that chemical goes on to tell the muscle to contract. Botulinum toxin actually stops this process. It prevents the release of this chemical from the nerve endings and as a result it gives rise to paralysis or weakness of the muscle, depending on the dose. The toxin attaches itself to the nerve terminals; it is something like ingested by the nerve terminal and then within the nerve cell it exerts its action to prevent the release of the substance called acetylcholine.

About the history of the toxin I think full credit has to be given to Alan Scott, who collaborated with the bacteriologist Edward Shantz. They worked together in the development of the toxin. Alan Scott is an ophthalmologist in San Francisco. He had been always longing to develop a method to replace surgery to treat a condition called strabismus, which is a condition of crossed eyes in children. In these children the eyes actually look in different directions, and the way to help them is to cut away one muscle that pulls the eye to one side and therefore the eyes can be restored to look straight ahead.

This procedure, he thought, might be replaced by an injection of a substance which could temporarily weaken the muscle. As the child grows up, the condition may be self-correcting, so if they are left with a normal muscle they probably will end up better. He had been working on that, and in 1973 in a publication we found out that this botulinum toxin A had been able to do that. That is, the substance is quite safe. It does not produce any generalized bad reactions. It does not produce any local reactions, and it can also give rise to a rather predictable weakness for a period of time, ranging from several months up to eight months in the monkey. With that he worked on to actually apply it in the human, and in 1980 he made the first publication of its use as an alternative to surgery in children, and he was quite successful with that.

The story would have just ended there, but there's another condition called blepharospasm. This condition, now classified as a neurological condition, is a focal dystonia. But because the symptoms occur in the eyelids, most patients go to see eye doctors because the eyes are blinking involuntarily. They think they have conjunctivitis or something wrong with the eyes. The eye doctors at first probably won't know what it is. The term *blepharospasm* is just a non-specific descriptive term.

The ophthalmologist Alan Scott, and other people too, then thought about the application of this toxin. They started injecting the muscles around the eyes and found out that it was useful. With the publication of these results it became clear that the drug can work for neurological conditions. From then on other neurologists started to think about the use of this toxin in other forms of focal dystonia, including the commonest form, neck dystonia. At that time three centers in North America started at the same time—in alphabetical order, Baylor College (Texas), Columbia University (New York), and our University of British Columbia (Vancouver)—all started at about the same time. The three leading people were Joseph Jankovic, Stanley Fahn, who later delegated all the work to Mitchell Brin, and Donald Calne of our center, who later on delegated this work to me. So these were the original people who can probably take the full credit for the development of the toxin to its use generally.

Would you say more about blepharospasm? How do you diagnose it, and how do you actually get the botulinum toxin to the right muscles?

Blepharospasm is actually the second commonest form of dystonia, and it is associated with oromandibular dystonia—that is, dystonic movements of the jaw, which is called Meige syndrome in North America. I always say that because Marsden in England tries to call it Brueghel's syndrome because he discovered a picture drawn by Brueghel in the 17th century of someone who actually looks ... the subject in the painting is displaying Meige syndrome. He tried to call it Brueghel's syndrome, but at international meetings nobody actually paid attention and that name has not gained any popularity.

With blepharospasm, the onset is usually insidious as a local irritation. Some people say that they have excessive tearing, some may have a sense of dryness of the eye—quite variable. Sunlight can aggravate it, anxiety can aggravate it. The severity can range from very mild—that is, not really very bothersome—to the eyes being constantly closed and patients can go and register themselves as blind.

We need to examine the patient very carefully and to rule out any local eye pathology. They may actually have conjunctivitis. After ruling all this out, we make a diagnosis of blepharospasm, but we always think about underlying causes, like neuroleptic drugs—drugs used for psychiatry that can produce funny combinations of dystonia and eye-blinking—that can be one of them. Wilson's disease is a copper-metabolism problem, which can present with dystonia but rarely just with blepharospasm. It's usually associated with other forms of dystonia, but we always think about this because it's a treatable condition. Most of the symptoms can be reversible. Other conditions should usually be very self-evident from clinical examination, and after excluding all these causes we call the condition *essential blepharospasm.*

Treatment available includes all medications, usually not very satisfactory again, as in all forms of dystonia. Surgery is always an alternative treatment in all kinds of dystonia. In the eyes it consists of cutting the muscles around the eyelids away. It can involve cutting the nerve fibers going to the eyelid muscle as well. But all these surgeries can be quite disfiguring, and they can affect normal function of eye closure, etc., so it is not very popular and reserved for extremely bad cases.

But of course botulinum toxin is now a very effective treatment and has replaced all forms of treatment. The injections themselves are quite simple. The injection technique can vary from center to center. This is our approach: we put just five injections around the eyelid muscle, but in other centers they may put it in different areas, some in three, some give seven, and the record number I've seen is seventeen around the eyes. The thing about this injection is that there is really no right way, and there's really no wrong way of doing it. The key is to pick up the correct muscle. No matter how many injections you give to the muscle, if you treat the correct muscle, then that's it. You're doing the right thing. But of course you also have to weigh against the patient's comfort level. In the face, eye-blinking is really very simple because there's only one muscle to think about. Nothing can go wrong with it. There are no other muscles to consider there.

You said you also use botulinum toxin with neck dystonia. But of course there are many more muscles in the neck than around the eye. Don't you have to use a lot more toxin in the neck? And what about side-effects of larger doses?

The side-effects of botulinum-toxin injection include generalized side-effects. Some patients may complain of some malaise after one injection, but this may not recur after the second injection. Interestingly, in one of our very early double-blind studies in 1986, when we injected the patients with a placebo—that is, with a blank injection—they also had those feelings of general tiredness, maybe a little spike of fever afterwards, and so on, so we believe that most of the generalized side-effects are probably not directly related to the botulinum-toxin injection.

But more pertinent to the injection would be local side-effects due to the traumatic injury, like local pain at the site of the injections. Some patients may complain of weakness of the neck. This is usually not very bad neck weakness, just some degree of weakness so that they notice it when they really want to exercise it. That is, they may have weakness lifting the head up when they bend forward but not affecting their daily activities.

Dysphagia, or swallowing problems, can occur, and this is extremely strange because we have seen so many patients, treated them all along with exactly the same technique and same dosages, and once in a while they will say that they have some dysphagia. Now this occurs in about 5% of injections and about 14% of patients. Sometimes it may recur in the same patient, and sometimes it may occur in patients who have never had it before.

I must say that we have not come across any allergic response to the botulinum-toxin injections.

There are lots of controversies in the application of it. First, there has been heated argument in international meetings about how to decide on the amount of toxin to be given to one muscle. How should we give it? Should we inject in one single bolus, or should we divide it into many, many different small injections—say, fifty units? Should we inject it in one spot of fifty or ten spots of five units? That's still controversial and still arguable, but so far our centre has been adopting a technique of trying to inject the least number of sites, limited by the volume.

We usually don't want to inject a big volume of substance into a single place because that's much more traumatic. That produces reactive bleeding, and the blood itself may somehow inactivate the toxin, and therefore we don't want to produce too much trauma by giving a large bolus. Again, we don't want to give too large a number of injections because it causes more pain. Therefore, the compromise is that we give a reasonable size of injection into one single area, usually 0.25 cc into one single area. That is one 100-unit vial of toxin: if you dilute it into one cc you divide it into four sites. And therefore for one muscle, if you need fifty mouse units, we would inject into two places only. (A mouse unit is defined as the lethal dose fifty for the mice. It sounds a little cruel, but if you inject one mouse unit into 100 mice of the same size—something like an 18- to 20-gram special strain of mouse—fifty of them will die. This is what we call one unit.)

In some other centres they do it in eight different sites for a particular muscle. I've heard people doing about thirty injections around the neck in different centres. Personally, I really don't see the logic behind many sites and small doses, especially if you want to inject a muscle called the splenius capitis. About 70% of that muscle is covered by another muscle, and if you really want to do multiple injections in that muscle, I don't know how you can do it without actually doing it blindly through another muscle. From the diagram drawn by the other centres who advocate multiple-site injections, in the splenius capitis they're still doing two or three injections only, limited by the availability of the surface anatomy, and therefore they are actually not practicing multiple-site injection in all the muscles.

Concerning frequency of injections, how soon should you do another treatment if it doesn't work? We have always been very conservative. We never wanted to treat the patients very frequently because we understand that it is a chronic condition. It takes time for the patient to develop the symptoms, and therefore we should be more patient and aim at a better result in the long run. If you really want to get quick results, you might want to inject a patient once, have them come back two weeks later, if it is not working, give them more, and so on and build it up accordingly. But the disadvantage is that you are easily overdosing the patient. You are easily giving them too many and too frequent injections, and theoretically it can increase the chance of producing antibodies, so in the long run the patients can develop a resistance to the treatment. Therefore, they may do more harm than good in that sense. According to our practice, we never inject the patients more frequently than once every nine weeks. This comes from previous experience.

We had the chance of treating patients with generalized dystonia with much higher doses and more frequently, and four of them developed antibodies and resistance to the toxin. Luckily, this does not happen with our patients with neck dystonia and other forms of focal dystonia because we have not been injecting them very frequently and we have not been giving them very high doses.

Dystonia is a very interesting syndrome in that sometimes you can have very complex patterns of movement, but sometimes only one or two muscles may be doing it while many other muscles are actually trying to compensate for the action or they are just triggered or associated movement. Therefore, sometimes if you can get the key muscles—just one or two of them—it may stop all the movements altogether.

If you start to be impatient, get one or two muscles, and then two weeks later get more and more, you may be actually cutting away those secondary, overactive muscles. I think we generally achieve better results if the patient comes back for the second or third time.

The dose of botulinum toxin: again, people talk about how many units are necessary for useful treatment. I don't think that is very meaningful because it really depends on the number of muscles involved. The more muscles the patient has involved in dystonia the higher the total dose would be. It probably makes more sense to talk about dose per muscle to be used. Right now, we are looking at something like fifty to seventy-five mouse units per muscle, though of course for the bigger muscles we may be using up to 100 mouse units.

These doses are actually very similar in different centres right now. We usually treat the patient with a dose that would be considered low in other centres, but we keep the dose unchanged usually when the patients come back. Normally, after one treatment the muscle would shrink down when it is not used any more because of the blockage, and after several months it will grow back but it is not yet back to its original size after three months. It usually takes six months for a muscle to regain its original power and original size. So three months later, when they come back, the muscle is still smaller than what it used to be. Keeping the dose unchanged would actually mean a relative increase in the dose for the same muscle, and therefore we are increasing the dose like that, that is, keeping the dose number unchanged but just giving the same dose into the smaller muscles, leaving a practical increase in dose.

You mentioned surgery in connection with blepharospasm. Is surgery ever useful in giving a patient relief from the twisting of neck muscles?

We are just trying to achieve about 70 to 80% weakness in the muscle. We never want to paralyze or take the muscle away completely because taking it away completely would be something which simulates surgery, which we don't want to do. The brain is a pretty smart organ. If you cut away the muscles, somehow the brain will tell the other muscles to do the same thing. There are about 55 muscles around the neck, including the head. If you cut away two or three muscles, the brain can always tell other muscles in the neck to do the same thing. That's why surgery works very well initially, and after a variable period of time, ranging from three months to a year, the patient could have a recurrence of the condition. And you just can't go in again and again and cut all the muscles away.

The good thing about botulinum toxin is that it's a dynamic process. Firstly, you don't take away the muscle completely and therefore you're fooling the brain. You let the brain know that the muscle is still there. It's still doing what you want to do, although it's not strong enough. If you inject too much into the muscle, you're killing the muscle, taking it completely away, and then the brain may know.

So botulinum-toxin injections work quite well with at least two forms of dystonia—affecting the eyes and the neck. What's your experience with using it for the other types of dystonia?

For oromandibular dystonia, one component of it involves the jaws. The jaw can remain clenched all the time. That's called jaw-closing dystonia. Botulinum-toxin injections have been very successful in treating it. Two big muscles here are the masseter and temporalis, both attached to the lower jaw. When they are active, they clench the jaws really tight. Injections of these muscles is very easy. You can see them. You can feel them. You can grab hold of them and put the needle in and inject the toxin. This has become very effective.

More difficult to treat is jaw-opening dystonia—that is, the mouth remains open all the time. Because the muscle is actually behind a piece of bone, it is more difficult to get at. The only hole we have to go through to the muscle is called the mandibular notch. This notch is more prominent when it is open. If you take this piece of bone away, it will expose a muscle called the lateral pterygoid muscle, which is lying right behind the bone. So if you go through a hole there, put a needle in about one inch deep, you would get at this muscle. Unfortunately, besides the lateral pterygoid, there is another muscle called the medial pterygoid, which is more difficult to get at. You need to go through the mouth to get into that muscle. I don't feel comfortable doing it. If necessary, I will ask my ear-nose-and-throat colleague to do it.

Then, we come to the condition of spasmodic dysphonia, which is a condition that involves vocal cords. It's a very interesting condition because patients can have a normal voice and they may be able to sing and shout relatively easily, but when they start talking it's very difficult. Most of them would find whispering much better. They whisper much more easily.

Spasmodic dysphonia can be subdivided into the adductor variety and the abductor variety. *Adductor* is the Latin term for bringing together. That is, the vocal cords are tight and they are brought together. Therefore, the voice sounds very high-pitched and strained. In this variety, the speech would be somewhat like this [speaks with strained sound]. It sounds very painful but in fact they are not in pain. It sounds agonizing but in fact they are frustrated. So this group of patients, when you ask them to give a long and loud eeee, like this, you can make the movements quite easily. They will say eeee [speaks with a more strained sound] and it'll stop. It becomes higher and higher and then stops. This is the adductor variety all right. This group of patients is much more common and they respond much better to botulinum-toxin injections.

Another group of spasmodic dysphonia patients does the opposite thing: the vocal cords are pulled apart so that they leak air all the time. When they talk, they sound something like this [talks with panting sound], as if they are short of breath. This is the abductor variety. If you ask them to say a long and loud eeee, it'll be eeee [makes breathy vowel sound] and it will be just sounding like air rushing out. This group of patients is much more difficult to treat, although they are much rarer.

If we look at the muscles around the vocal cords from the top, two muscles pull the vocal cords together, and therefore, if they are tight, they will produce a very tight tension of the voice. This can be injected through the front, through the skin and a membrane. You can get at these muscles quite easily. For this I would strongly advocate the use of EMG [electromyography] because you really need to know that you are in this muscle because there is really no guidance. When you ask the patient to activate the voice and you see the spikes [on the EMG screen], you squirt in the toxin and then you are home.

Injecting these muscles is relatively safe. The side-effects are that, if you weaken these muscles too much, the vocal cords will actually move apart and you would end up with a breathy voice like the other variety. It's usually transient. You have a little choking for a short time, but that is not very dangerous. The dangerous thing to do is that, if you treat the opposite group by injecting the muscles in the back, that pulls the vocal cords apart. But if you overdo it, the vocal cords would collapse together and it would block the breathing; therefore, it can be quite dangerous. People are advocating the use of toxin on one side only for this group of patients, and people still report varying degrees of success with the abductor variety.

Then comes the limb dystonia—writer's cramp, hand dystonia, upper-limb dystonia, and lower-limb dystonia. In hand dystonia, I think the use of botulinum toxin is really quite limited by the fact that it may reduce the dystonia but it may produce too much weakness in the same muscles which are important in normal function. We may easily correct the abnormal posture, but most of the time we do not restore a lot of functions in the hand.

In one of our patients, the wrist was always twisted at a right angle, and after botulinum-toxin injections, it was quite straight—close to 180 degrees. But the patient did not have any important functions restored in that hand, although the patient felt much more comfortable.

Foot dystonia is much more worthwhile treating. If it is very difficult for the heel to touch the ground, the foot becomes inverted—faces inward. All we need to do is to get at a muscle at the top and reduce the dystonia sufficiently so that the patient can have the foot flat on the ground. In one extreme example a young boy was presenting with foot dystonia in both legs. The toes were always pointed. The dystonia started at the age of seven. After a short time he had to use a wheelchair all the time because he couldn't even stand. He was wheelchair-bound for two years before he came to us. After injection of the muscle bilaterally, slowly after a year he could put his foot flat on the ground and he could walk. Another year later he could run. So it can help the patient that much by just treating foot dystonia.

For hand dystonia it's much less useful. I only do it for specific indications. That depends upon how much it affects the patient. Some patients can have dystonia of the hand so bad that it is bent all the time, and they have a lot of hygienic problems. Seeing patients with infection increases. This is really worthwhile treating because after the injections they can open the hand, they can clean it, and infection clears up. Some of these patients may just want the hand to be straight so that they can shake hands with other people or hold the hand of a granddaughter.

If only the back muscles are involved, then it's easy. You use as much botulinum toxin as you like and weaken the muscles in the back sufficiently so that the dystonia is corrected. But unfortunately, in many patients the muscles in front of the vertical columns may be involved too, and these muscles are difficult. Most of the patients with generalized dystonia may have a curved body and they may arch forward. That means that the muscles in the front are involved, and these muscles you really cannot get at—not through the front and through many organs, nor through the back. Frequently, they have abdominal muscles involved as well.

Dystonia: The Disease That Distorts

It's very complex, and again we don't really know how much toxin we can use in a single patient in a single setting. So far we have not gone over 400. In our centre we have always been very conservative. I've never gone over 400, and in the neck I've never gone over 300.

So the conclusion in dystonia is that in individual areas it seems to be very successful in facial dystonia. In ormandibular dystonia it is only successful in jaw-closing. In jaw-opening dystonia in selected cases it may work very well. For neck dystonia it's very helpful. Hand dystonia—again, in selected cases. Foot dystonia—always worthwhile going into. Back dystonia—it depends on the direction of pull: if it is to one side and back, then one may contemplate doing the back paraspinal muscle, but if the twist is to one side and forward, chances are that you will not be able to help the patient a lot.

This also applies to generalized dystonia; you may need to pick one or two areas that affect the patient most and then pick out those areas to inject. I'm currently treating quite a few generalized-dystonia patients in the limbs, just trying to correct the posture to make them functionally more useful because some of them are in the electrically operated wheelchair. Correcting elbow joints, for example, can help them rest their hand more comfortably on the switch and they can manipulate the switches.

Is botulinum toxin useful for any disorders besides dystonia?

Because of the success in dystonia, botulinum toxin is also tried in other conditions like spasticity, multiple sclerosis, cerebral palsy, stroke conditions, tremor, and a whole lot of applications. That is all coming from research in dystonia. The approved [by the Food and Drug Administration] applications in North America remain strabismus— that is the cross-eyed—and facial injections— blepharospasm, hemifacial spasm, and other facial movements. But scientifically it has already been accepted as the most effective treatment for neck dystonia, jaw-closing dystonia, and the adductor variety of vocal-cord dystonia. It remains investigational [as of 1993] in writer's cramp and limb dystonia, trunk dystonia, and the abductor variety of spasmodic dysphonia—the vocal-cord dystonia.

There is no doubt that injection of botulinum toxin leads to muscle weakness. Secondly, after the weakness of the muscle, it will correct incorrect posture in most cases if you get the correct muscle. But here is something that we need to think about: how do we help the patient by weakening those muscles? This is the question that a physician who does the injections should always ask himself. Am I going to help the patient by weakening this muscle?

You mentioned antibodies to botulinum toxin. Is there any research on other types of substances that can work as an acetylcholine blocker?

That was originally work of Alan Scott. He has studied four of the most eligible substances at that time, including a snake poison. All these are very potent toxins to muscles that can stop muscle actions, but he found either that the drugs were inducing too much local reaction or that they are too toxic and too permanent.

The issue about botulinum toxin is not that it does not work long enough, because its effects individually at the neuromuscular junction can be said to be permanent but the patient actually recovers by his own regeneration. So it is probably more dependent on the patient's own regeneration process, which governs the duration of effectiveness. I don't think we can get any toxin that can work longer—a permanent substance. But if you want to get a more potent toxin to induce more paralysis of a muscle, this is something that we don't want to do. We don't really want to kill the muscle completely. So far I think botulinum toxin remains still the ideal substance.

You said that botulinum toxin usually has to be injected every two or three months. Do the effects ever last longer than that?

So far it has been found to be still effective for at least nine years, but that's the longest experience that we have, and that's all we can tell you. On the other hand, there has been a proposal about developing a substance which may delay nerve regeneration, and injected together with botulinum toxin, might delay that process. But it's only talking. I don't think anyone has come up with a substance like that yet. But that's another approach which may prolong the action.

The long-term effect of the toxin is still very, very unclear. You must understand that we are really talking in terms of nanograms. With most therapeutic agents we talk about milligrams. A nanogram is a millionth of a gram. The amount is so small that it's really difficult to trace, and that small an amount I don't really know how much it can do to the body generally. The amount of the toxin injected in the body is so small nobody can effectively trace where the toxin goes.

I think that the lifetime accumulation of a patient starting at the age of 30 right up to the age of 70 is probably not going to be that much. And also right now there is no clinical evidence of generalized effect of the toxin, although some very sensitive EMG techniques have shown that it also affects the neuromuscular junction—that is, the junction where the toxin works—in areas that are very far away from the site of injection. But that is very much unknown. We don't know what it actually means so far. There's a little worry there but not a major worry. I must say that people are keeping their eye on and monitoring all these problems. No problems have so far come up.

Chapter 7

Seeking Answers from Medical Research

The more we explore the varied and often complex symptoms of dystonia, the more apparent is our ignorance of its causes. With symptoms that seem to come from nowhere—from no readily identifiable cause or circumstance—we are left with questions that have no present answers.

In the attempt to find those answers, the Belzberg family of Vancouver, British Columbia, began the Dystonia Medical Research Foundation in 1976. As its name implies, the Foundation's principal purpose is to support research into this puzzling phenomenon. As of 1995, $13 million gathered by the Foundation has supported research into the causes of and treatments for dystonia. The Foundation's Scientific Advisory Board, comprised of leading scientists and physicians, reviews proposals from all over the world and recommends to the Foundation's Board of Directors those most deserving of funds.

For a number of years, the National Institutes of Health (NIH) has increasingly included dystonia among its research priorities. This has helped increase the momentum and intensity of study, raising expectations that answers to some of the most significant questions may be forthcoming.

Dystonia: The Disease That Distorts

Among the most promising recent research directions of the Dystonia Medical Research Foundation are studies on the genetic basis for dystonia. Dr. Laurie Ozelius, a genetic researcher at Massachusetts General Hospital, has spent the past eleven years in the laboratory of Dr. Xandra Breakefield, the researcher who originated this work.

You are working in one of the principal American laboratories associated with genetic research on dystonia. Recent newspaper and magazine articles have suggested that genetic research may reveal causes of many diseases. Is dystonia one of them? Please explain whether and how genetic research might help us understand what causes dystonia and how to treat it better.

Because some forms of dystonia are inherited, family studies should help us to clarify the number of different genes involved in causing dystonia. Getting a handle on the different genes is important in terms of better classifying the different clinical subtypes of dystonia. Hopefully, if we can find some of these genes, this should increase our understanding of the mechanism of the disease and perhaps allow us to design more effective and better treatments.

Perhaps you should first explain what a gene is.

Our bodies are made up of millions of cells, and each of these cells has a central region called the nucleus. Within this nucleus are chromosomes, which contain information for all inherited traits—the color of your hair, the color of your eyes, your height, everything. We have 46 chromosomes—23 from our mother and 23 from our father. These chromosomes are made up of DNA, and a small segment of DNA that codes for an inherited trait is called a gene. There are thousands of these genes on every chromosome, and you can think of them as lined up like beads on a string. The chromosomes come in pairs—one set from your mom and one set from your dad. This means that for each gene you have two copies. There are at least 100 thousand genes spread out across all of these chromosomes.

How exactly do you go about finding the one gene or genes associated with dystonia?

We use something called positional cloning. Using this technique we try to find our gene based on its position on the chromosome. To do this we have to have markers that are evenly spaced along each chromosome. A marker is a DNA sequence whose transmission can be observed because it has a polymorphism, or variation. Just like genes, a marker can be passed from a parent to a child, and there are two copies of each marker, one from each parent.

How do these markers actually help locate a gene?

When two markers are close together on the same chromosome, they are inherited together. What we look for are variations that show one pattern in all affected members of the family and a different pattern in the unaffected members of the family. If we find a marker that behaves in this manner, then we know that it is located close to or linked to the disease gene. Because we know the chromosomal location of the marker, we then know the position of the disease gene.

In the case of early-onset dystonia, we found markers from the tip of the long arm of chromosome 9 to be linked or close to the disease gene in one large, non-Jewish family. Subsequently, we found that markers from this same region were also linked in families of Jewish origin, suggesting the same gene was involved in their dystonia. In both cases, the markers that were linked spanned a fairly large region that probably contained over a thousand genes. We were down from hundreds of thousands of genes to around a thousand genes, but this was still too many genes to sort through to find our one gene of interest.

Much of your research has been focused on one group of people from eastern Europe— Ashkenazi Jews. Why is that group of such interest in narrowing down your search for that one gene?

Early-onset dystonia is at least ten times more frequent among the Ashkenazi Jews. That is probably because the Ashkenazi Jews tend to intermarry and are thus more related to each other. We wondered if all the affected individuals in the Ashkenazi-Jewish population might be related to a single ancestor, who actually passed the disease on to all of the Ashkenazi Jews who have the disease today. If this were true, it could help us to get closer to the disease gene. This phenomenon is called *linkage disequilibrium* or *allele association*. It means that the markers that stay with the disease gene over hundreds of years are the markers that are the very closest. In practical terms, what we want to find is some kind of variation that is more common among unrelated, affected Ashkenazi Jews than among unaffected Ashkenazi Jews. When we looked at the linked markers, one of these showed this association. We found that 69% of affected chromosones had a common variation, while less than 2% of control chromosomes showed that specific variation. As we generated more markers near the original marker, we found that they all had one variation (which we call an *allele*) that was much more frequent among the affected chromosomes than on the unaffected chromosomers. This suggested that they were all very close to the disease gene.

When we take all of these associated alleles together, we call it a haplotype. This haplotype marks the chromosome on which the original mutation occurred in the Ashkenazi population hundreds of years ago. What this means is that, when the mutation occurred, those variations were already present on the chromosome. Thus, everybody who is descended from that person and received the disease gene also has those particular variations. This is why we can do genetic testing on the Ashkenazi-Jewish population. We don't have to have the disease gene; we can just look at these markers that we know are very close— and look for the particular variations that make up the associated haplotype. If someone has the haplotype, then we are pretty sure they carry the disease gene.

Is it only speculation about the nature of the mutation or what might have been the cause?

We don't know the type of mutation or its cause. It just arose somehow.

Back to linkage disequilibrium. How exactly does linkage disequilibrium, or allele association, get you closer to the gene?

The vast majority of the Ashkenazi patients have this intact haplotype; they have the whole thing—2, 8, 16, 12, 4 [numbers of variations associated with the markers]. But there are some individuals who only retain a portion of this haplotype. Those are the individuals that we want to concentrate on because, even though they don't have all of the associated variations, they still have the disease. Thus the portion of the haplotype that is retained in all of these individuals also has to contain the disease gene. They all retain the 16 variation; thus the gene is somehwere around the 16 allele. The region around the 16 variation contains probably about 10 genes and is small enough to try and clone.

How do you clone genes?

We use what we call libraries to clone genes. You can think of these libraries just like your local library, except that these libraries contain books with pieces of chromosome 9 in them. What we want to do is check out all the books that contain our region of interest. When we find these books, we then look for more markers in the books to try to make our region smaller, and we also start to look for the genes that are in these books. We are now trying to assess these four, five, or six genes that are left in the region to find out which one is actually the disease gene.

Even though you haven't actually located and studied that disease gene, you're calling it the DYT1 gene, aren't you?

Correct.

Will that genetic information about early-onset, generalized dystonia have application to other kinds of dystonia in people who are not Jewish?

The real answer to that is that we don't know. But we have some evidence to suggest that at least some focal dystonias might have something to do with this gene. There are some families, both Jewish and non-Jewish, where there's an affected child with generalized dystonia but then there'll be a relative that only has a focal dystonia. But we know that they carry the same gene. So that means that this gene—DYT1—can somehow manifest itself and show the clinical symptoms of focal dystonia. Why one person will get generalized dystonia and another person will get focal dystonia, when they have the exact same gene and presumably the exact same mutation, we don't know. Whether there are other genes that are protective or genes that make you susceptible or perhaps environmental factors that come into play, we don't know.

We do know that dopa-responsive dystonia, or Segawa's dystonia, has a genetic basis, don't we?

There was controversy over whether hereditary-progressive dystonia, or Segawa's dystonia, and dopa-responsive dystonia (DRD) were actually the same disease or not, but then they were both linked to the same region on chromosome 14, indicating that they are the same disease. Recently the Japanese found the gene for this form of dystonia. It is called GTP cyclohydrolase 1. They tested this gene in some of their patients and found several mutations in it that knocked out the function of the gene. This is one form of dystonia that actually is treatable with very low doses of l-dopa, the same drug that they use to treat Parkinson's disease. You give this drug to these patients and they are pretty much cured.

Why did it prove possible to discover what that gene was—not only the location but the gene itself—when it's not possible with other forms of dystonia yet?

Well, because this form of dystonia is so treatable, and from this treatment some clues can be garnered as to the mechanism behind DRD. The treatment suggests that the dopamine pathway is involved—how you get from tyrosine to dopamine. This pathway is very well studied, very well known, because Parkinson's disease involves this same pathway. Lots of research has been done on Parkinson's disease, a lot more than dystonia.

When an interesting candidate gene of known function (the GTP-cyclohydrolsase-1 gene) mapped onto chromosome 14, it was only a matter of testing this one gene whose function and sequence were already known. This gene—GTPCH1—is involved in the dopamine pathway. Thus far, none of the genes in the DYT1 region look like any known gene, and there are no real clues from the pathology, biochemistry, or pharmacology of primary dystonias to tell us what kind of gene we should be looking for. Therefore, we need to test each gene that is in our critical region for any kind of change that is specific to the disease.

———

One of Laurie Ozelius's colleagues in these genetic studies is Patricia Kramer of Oregon Health Sciences University. A population geneticist, Dr. Kramer is also presently a member of the Foundation's Scientific Advisory Board.

What can you add to Laurie Ozelius's explanation of research that links the "classic" (early-onset generalized) dystonia to the DYT1 gene?

The next step of the work that needs to be done is to study adult-onset, focal dystonias. We haven't cloned the DYT1 gene but it will be done and it will be done soon. In the meantime we've neglected the adult-onset dystonias, and that's what we're trying to make some advances on. We don't know very much.

The early-onset forms of classic dystonia in both Ashkenazi-Jewish and non-Jewish families for the most part all appear to be due to mutations in the DYT1 gene on chromosome 9, clearly all autosomal dominant. (Pure and simple autosomal-dominant inheritance means this: the affected individual has a 50% chance of giving the **disease** gene to any offspring and a 50% chance of giving the **nondisease** gene to any offspring.)

There are at least two variant forms of early-onset dystonia that are not caused by the DYT1 gene on chromosome 9. In the late-onset dystonias, they all appear to be autosomal dominant with much reduced penetrance.

Please explain *penetrance.*

The additional glitch in dystonia is that this disease gene has reduced penetrance. Our estimate for dystonia is that the penetrance is reduced to 30 to 40%, meaning that, even if you inherit the gene from a parent, you only have 30 to 40% chance of manifesting symptoms of dystonia.

So you do have some evidence that late-onset dystonias may be caused by some gene other than DYT1?

It's not clear whether these late-onset forms are due to mutations in the DYT1 gene or in other genes or are not genetic at all. There are a couple of variant forms of late-onset dystonia. One is a form that is rapid-onset—sometimes overnight. It's clearly autosomal dominant and not linked to the DYT1 gene on chromsome 9; it is a different gene, not found yet. There is an X-linked form of dystonia with Parkinson-like symptoms that is on the X chromosome; in other words, there's no father-to-son transmission. [Females carry two X chromosomes; males carry one X and one Y chromosome.] But this is pretty much localized to the Philippines.

We know that those individuals who carry the haplotype for early-onset generalized dystonia have a mutation in the DYT1 gene. We don't know what causes the dystonia in those individuals who don't carry the haplotype. Many of these individuals are familial cases, so we assume that there is a genetic basis for their dystonia. Some of them may be caused by different mutations in the DYT1 gene, so the markers that they show would be different. Some of them may be caused by different genes altogether on different chromosomes. And certain cases are not genetic at all.

These studies are in their infancy and one of the reasons why is because in autosomal-dominant forms of focal dystonia the penetrance is probably even less than 20%, so you don't get very often huge families with many affected individuals. You might get a family with two, three, maybe four individuals. Those are very small families. That's why it's difficult to do genetic studies.

In one Swedish family at least 7 of 26 members are definitely affected with primarily blepharospasm and torticollis; one individual had arm dystonia. The age of onset is between the ages of 14 and 50, which is essentially later-adolescent, adult-onset dystonia. We have excluded this family from being linked to the DYT1 gene, and this is our first strong hold on feeling that there are other genes than the DYT1 that are important in the later-onset dystonias.

What should people who have a form of late-onset focal dystonia do that might help to help genetic researchers like you get the information you need?

I think that the most important thing is to talk with as many family members as possible just to make it known. I'm not a clinician so I don't deal with patients in a clinical setting, but I've talked with a number of clinicians.

One clinician in particular was telling me he wasn't convinced that there was much of a genetic basis in late-onset dystonia. For the people he saw in the BOTOX clinic, family history never seemed to come up with too much. But the more he listened to me the more he said, "Well, maybe she's got something." That happened after he was talking to a young man who I think had blepharospasm, asking him about family history. No, there was no history at all. While he was in the clinic being treated, the young man noticed another patient who had torticollis. He then said, "Oh, gosh, that person ... my dad has that same thing." The clinician said, "Well, but don't you understand that this is probably also dystonia?" So it turned out his father and an uncle had torticollis and he had blepharospasm.

The most important thing at this point—particularly in the late-onset forms where you really don't have pure-breeding torticollis or pure-breeding blepharospasm or even spasmodic dysphonia—is that an affected family member doesn't necessarily have to have exactly the same kind of dystonia as you do.

What seem to you to be the likely pathways or directions of dystonia research in the next generation?

I think one of the most exciting things is going to be—once the gene is cloned—to determine what it actually does and to see what it tells us about neuroscience in general. It's obviously a gene that nobody's identified yet, just as there are many, many genes that haven't been identified yet.

Once it has been identified, we need to see its part in the nervous system. This goes beyond its particular relationship to dystonia. We often say *the DYT1 gene*, meaning it perhaps is a gene which causes dystonia. In its "normal" condition this gene has a function, and it's a mutation in the gene that causes dystonia. Once we realize what its primary function is and how that relates to the rest of our nervous system, this will make a valuable contribution to neuroscience in the name of dystonia. I think that's going to be a fascinating thing to do. Once that gene is cloned and particular parts of it are identified in terms of what controls what, you can then induce mutations in rats and see how that is manifested. So it could become a gene that's important, that's very broadly important.

Clearly, from a patient's point of view, the most important thing in this generation, once that gene is identified, is how it will lead to beneficial treatment. Cure is probably several generations down the road because of the amount of time it takes to actually work on protocols to introduce this into the human system and to determine clearly how that's going to affect treatment.

In terms of sporadic cases of dystonia, once that gene is identified and we know what it does, it could have implications for more effective treatment, even in people with non-genetic forms of dystonia. Just because somebody might have a mutation of a particular gene that causes that person to have dystonia doesn't mean that somebody who has dystonia from a non-genetic form might not benefit from treatments derived from the genetics.

I think those are the two most exciting areas in the next ten years. I think we're going to find a number of what you might call minor dystonia genes. In other words, they cause certain forms of dystonia, but it's going to be a sub-set of individuals here and a sub-set of individuals there. That's no less important for that sub-set of individuals. That's going to be a little slower, but I think that's probably going to take off. It's going to take us much less time because of improvements in molecular and statistical and computer technologies to find genes.

I know that most researchers would say that they aren't adequately funded, no matter how much money they have. How close would you say dystonia research of the kind that is now feasible is to being adequately funded? What's the gap between what we need and what we have presently? I ask this of you because you're a member of the Scientific Advisory Board of the

Dystonia Medical Research Foundation, so you see all of the proposals that come in.

Though there hasn't always been a lot of money, it seems as though, when it's clear that a particular line of work is necessary and being done accurately, the Dystonia Medical Research Foundation finds the money. They may not always find enough, but they find the money.

I'll speak now in terms of looking for other dystonia genes and the adult-onset forms. Collecting family data is very, very expensive. You've got phone calls. You've got to bring people in to be examined or send out a team to examine them. You have to collect blood and get that blood transported. It takes a lot of time and it takes a lot of money. You have to pay a clinician, as well as a genetics counselor. So, yes, if God came to me in a dream and said, "What kind of study would you like to do and how much money do you need?" it would be a lot more than is actually available.

But when I look at what has been done so far and the amount of money that has been spent on it, I think it's been very efficiently done. And that's because many of the people who have been primarily involved have some sort of a vested interest in the research: who have loved ones who are afflicted. That in itself is enough to inspire. So the mission of the Foundation I think has inspired the work.

———

Dr. Joel Perlmutter of Washington University (St. Louis) heads a research effort that complements work in genetics but studies dystonia from a different perspective. His work, first supported by the Mattie Lou Koster Benign Essential Blepharospasm Foundation, is now supported by a major grant from NIH.

The research on dystonia that you are doing at Washington University does not involve genetics. What is it called?

The name of the grant is "PET Investigations of Dystonia." The research questions specifically are twofold: 1) Do people with dystonia have a change or a difference in their dopamine-receptor binding compared to people without dystonia? and 2) Do people with dystonia that affects the hand, compared to people with dystonia that affects predominantly the eyelids, have a difference in the location of their maximal dopamine-receptor binding in a part of the brain called the putamen?

Let's explore those questions in a minute. First, though, what is a PET scan and how does it work?

To do a PET (or, positron emission tomography) scan, which is really a way of looking at how the brain functions, we need to have something to monitor with that scanner. And what we monitor or measure that gets into the brain are radioisotopes. These radioisotopes are short-lived, which means they don't hang around very long. For example, one of them that we inject is a radioactive form of oxygen attached to water. The radioactive form has a half life of two minutes. We have two cyclotrons and a linear accelerator here at Washington University that produce these isotopes for us. When we inject one of these things, it's like getting an X-ray exposure, but it's fairly small.

Here's what we do when you lie down in our scanner. We make this mask that molds right to your face and helps to hold your head in place for the whole study. Holding your head still for one of these studies is quite key. You get into that scanner and we make these kinds of pictures, giving a slice through the brain. The PET image appears to show the structure, but it's really very different. We're showing how the brain is functioning. So if in fact we take a picture of your brain in the PET with certain kinds of radioisotopes, we will see those parts of the brain that are actively doing something. If we have you opening and closing your hand during a PET scan, we'll see that part of the brain important for opening and closing the hand become more active. In that way we can map out the function and see how it works.

What part of the brain are you looking at in dystonia?

We think the inner parts—the basal ganglia—are important for control of smooth movement, and these areas of the brain are also connected by circuits to other areas that are important for movement as well in a more direct fashion. We would like to look at how these different parts of the brain are functioning in dystonia.

For example, in idiopathic dystonia—that's the kind in which we don't identify a specific cause—it's known that if we actually peek at the brain with an MRI [magnetic resonance imaging] scan or a CT [computed tomography] scan the brain indeed looks normal. It was about twelve or thirteen years ago we had a person who had an unusual kind of dystonia that affected just one side of the body and who also had a normal CT scan or MRI scan of the brain. But when we put him in the PET scanner we found a distinctly abnormally functioning part of the brain in the basal ganglia. That was one of the early clues that this part of the brain was involved with dystonia. Also, other people who had strokes occasionally in this area would sometimes develop dystonia.

Could we go back now to the first of your two research questions? What kinds of changes in the brains of people with dystonia are you studying?

In people who have idiopathic dystonia—not caused by a stroke or anything—the structures look normal. However, there were some clues in these forms of dystonia that there may be things not working so normally. For somebody whose head is twisting or eyes are squeezing shut, if they just touch themselves sometimes on the chin or between the eyes, that kind of sensory information may help relieve the twisting of the head or the squeezing of the eyelids shut. This suggests that somehow the brain-processing of this sensory information—turning it into a motion—might be different and important for causing the dystonia.

So we looked at how the brain processes sensory information in people with dystonia. We measured in the PET the blood flow to different parts of the brain. You see, blood flow is an indication of how much those brain nerve cells are working. We did that with the person lying at rest and while touching a vibrator to their hand. We did this in people who had dystonia just on one side of the body.

In a normal brain we can see a little spot that gets a marked increase in blood flow after stimulation. That's the part of the brain that's important for feeling and moving the hand. When we did it with somebody who had dystonia on the left side of the body and then touched the left hand, we found a diminished response—25 to 30% lower than what would happen in a brain without dystonia.

That response, however, occurred in the same location of the brain whether the person had dystonia or didn't have dystonia. It was just that the magnitude of that response was diminished. In fact, that abnormal dysfunction was on both sides of the brain, whether that side of the body had dystonia or not. Part of the reason may be some of the people we studied went on to develop dystonia on the other side of the body, but it could be a general phenomenon going on in the brain in addition to what you see outside. So we found abnormalities in the primary sensory-motor area of the brain in these people with dystonia.

So what? Who cares about these blood-flow responses in the brain? How does that help you get to the next step? And what is the next step?

It is to look at how these areas might be connected to the basal ganglia and how drugs or other maneuvers may alter these responses—return them to normal or if in fact these other areas are functioning abnormally so we can identify if the primary problem is because the basal ganglia is not letting this part of the brain work right.

This, then, must be where your second research question comes in.

The basal ganglia are connected to the cortex, where we've been looking at responses. Also, these parts of the brain use a chemical called dopamine as a chemical messenger to send messages between different nerve cells. Dopamine has been a very suspicious character over the years. Alterations of dopamine or blocking the effects of dopamine in some cases can produce dystonic postures. In some cases making alterations in dopamine seems to help people with dystonia. So it's kind of a suspicious story here. We want to try to sort that out.

And how might that be effective?

We had a person who had dystonia on one side of the body whose dystonia was markedly improved by small doses of dopa, which converts in the body to dopamine. So that was a dopa-responsive dystonia. When we did the vibration study on that person in the side that was abnormal—the right side where she had dystonia—the response in the brain in this person was markedly diminished in the left side of the brain. Vibrate the right hand that had dystonia: the left brain didn't respond normally. Vibrate her normal left side: her right brain responded normally. (The old brain's cross-eyed, you know. The right brain controls the left body.)

But when we gave her Sinemet, which has the dopa in it, her dystonia melted and now the response in her brain became normal. We think it's because the dopamine is acting as a chemical messenger and normalizing the circuitry that goes out to the motor-control part of the brain.

What specifically does dopamine do in the brain?

Dopamine gets released from a nerve and sends its message to the receiving nerve cell. When it does that, to make that message connect, it has to stick at a very specific spot called the receptor. This conveyance of information can get screwed up (that's a technical medical term) if this receptor is not functioning properly. So what we'd like to do is measure these dopamine receptors. We can do that in the PET scanner too.

We inject a radio-labelled chemical that goes directly to stick to that dopamine-receptor site—and there are different kinds of dopamine-receptor sites. We do a very specific one, identifying where it sticks and how sticky it is there. Then we see if there's a change in these dopamine receptors in people with dystonia—not only whether there's a change as far as too much or too little, but also—and this is the neat little part of it—whether the place where it sticks maximally is different for somebody who has dystonia that affects the eyes, like blepharospasm, compared to somebody who has dystonia that affects the hands, like writer's cramp. Is it different because this different part of the brain is organized by body part, perhaps? So if it's stickier in one place, maybe there'll be dystonia in the hand. If it's stickier in another place, maybe there'll be dystonia in the face. We hypothesize that but nobody knows that.

If we could start to understand the organization of these parts of the brain, that's a far further step toward getting an appropriate treatment when these parts of the brain go awry.

————

Dr. Joseph Tsui, whose experience in the treating dystonia with botulinum toxin is vast, as shown in Chapter 6, has taken still another complementary line of research.

Your dystonia center in Vancouver, B.C. has been a principal source of research on the use of botulinum toxin in treating dystonia. But now I understand that you are engaged in another kind of research.

What I've started doing is to have an epidemiological survey in British Columbia on the actual prevalence of dystonia. We can do it now because we have been very lucky in that we developed the botulinum-toxin program and we have been the only center in the area. So we can sort of proudly say that we are probably draining all the patients from the local area, not to mention people from other areas too. But if you want to do a good epidemiological study, there are limited ways. You can go to a door-to-door survey, which is very, very time-consuming. But now we have the advantage of people coming to us, and we have also for the past three years very successfully improved the awareness of dystonia around British Columbia.

And another thing that we can be proud of is that the average time taken for a patient to see doctor, from the beginning of symptoms to the diagnosis of dystonia, had been seven years, before we started the program. Right now, with the botulinum-toxin injections and with the educational program carried out for practitioners, this has been shortened to less than a year. So we are now picking up new cases much faster and therefore an epidemiological survey would probably be much more accurate.

We will interview all our patients from British Columbia, and we will definitely go into the family history in much greater detail. Very often when you see a patient and ask them "Any family with a similar illness?" they will just casually say "No." And then if you ask them again and again three or four more times as they come, they will say, "Now I remember that a distant uncle had something probably like a writing problem or shaking of the hand and so on." What I always ask them to do is to go back and look at the family album and pick out from there whether there are any people with a twisted neck, etc.

Now all these will be revisited and then we can probably have a better understanding of the family history of these patients. Now if the family history comes up to be significantly higher—because right now we find it to be very, very low in focal dystonia—we pick up all those families. We are now linked up with the medical-genetics people, and they can certainly try to identify a possible gene for the dystonia. Because if it turns out to be a genetic illness, then the approach of treatment will be completely different.

Now the other thing about especially torticollis, for example: I believe that it is a mixed bag of disease. Some may be hereditary. Some may be secondary—that is, environmental, caused by some medications—drugs. Some may be traumatic. There's a mixed bag of illness. From our survey, possibly we can categorize them into different groups and then identify the characteristics of these people. Because to each group the approach can be entirely different. The cure or the treatment can be entirely different. So these are the various aspects that our future research will be looking into.

How will your epidemiological study be tied to the molecular study that underlies genetic research?

The molecular biology aspect of it is tied to the epidemiological if something comes up—something like a genetic or hereditary component for focal dystonia, for example. Then the molecular biology would be able to set in for identification of the gene.

Will you collect blood samples?

Yes. We uniformly take a sample of blood from all the patients coming in, although not all will be analyzed, but we keep them in a safe place and the medical-genetics people can deal with them. Then when we take out indexed cases, these can be specifically studied. So this is a prospective study.

Now the other thing molecular biology can help is that the gene marker for generalized dystonia—on chromosome 9q—has been identified. This is a very important thing to identify because this sequence of events, if it is known, then the cure for dystonia would be much closer.

Many pathological studies—collections of brains—are also important because we suspect dystonia is a disorder of the basal ganglia. It has never been definitely proven. It has only been indirectly proven because of some rare cases of maybe a tumor or stroke in some parts of the brain. That produces something that is similar to dystonia, and that's how we infer from it. But from the previous pathological studies in dystonia, when the brains were examined they all looked normal. Those were from years ago. The staining technique and the knowledge of neurotransmitters were not as good as now. Now we have much more knowledge, but we have no brains. I don't really want the patient's brain, but it's a useful thing to get involved with. It may not help the patient immediately, but in future it can turn out to be very important.

Would it be fair to say that, as far as your perspective on research is concerned, we're still in the extremely early stages of understanding dystonia?

Yes. Extremely early.

Could you compare it with any other better known disease and place us in some sort of time relationship?

Now let's put it this way. For dystonia, we started off late. Research on dystonia really only started probably about ten years ago. And within ten years, we've come to the understanding of the nature of dystonia. We've come up with a rather effective symptomatic treatment for focal dystonia. All these accomplishments in the line of research would be considered as quick, although it may not seem so for the patient.

Look at Parkinson's disease: 1966 was the first publication of levadopa being helpful in Parkinson's disease. Ten years later we came up with another new drug which has been quite significant. And after that and up to now there hasn't been any more significant new discovery in therapeutics that would be comparable to those. Botulinum toxin is something that is comparable in dystonia to levadopa in Parkinson's disease, and that has occurred within ten years of focused research.

Now what I can foresee in dystonia is that, at least for the genetic group, genetic manipulation will be probably the future. I don't know how distant the future would be, but we must work along that line. But to get that going, one must understand how a gene expresses itself as dystonia. That's I think the ultimate line of research there.

———————

Just a few years ago, we sometimes referred to dystonia as an orphan disease—one that was neglected in comparison with such better known diseases as Parkinson's, cancer, cerebral palsy, and multiple dystrophy. But with the accelerated pace of research in the past ten years, the likelihood of identifying and cloning the gene or genes responsible for dystonia is now greatly increased, and effective treatments are perhaps a little less remote. Those whose muscles have been distorted by this perplexing disease can't yet relax and enjoy a normal life. But they have at least the consolation that dystonia is no longer an orphan in the scientific world, thanks to the Dystonia Medical Research Foundation and its thousands of committed volunteers.

Index

catheterize 99
cause 3, 8, 20-21, 32, 42, 86, 99, 104, 111,
    133-134, 138, 142-143, 145-146, 149-150, 156
cerebral palsy 37, 129, 159
cervical dystonia 10, 45, 62, 91, 106
charley horse 10
childhood 42
chiropractor 36
clostridium botulinum 112
Clozaril 55
Columbia University 58, 82, 84, 115
concentrate 91
congenital abnormality 106
conjunctivitis 14, 114, 116
contiguous body parts 43
    head and neck 43
    leg and trunk 43
    neck and trunk 43
cooking 74
Cooper, Dr. Irving S. 68-69, 71
coordination 20, 74, 75
cortex 108
cotton mouth 59
cramp 5, 6, 19, 20, 34, 46, 57, 106-108, 110,
    126, 129, 154
cranial dystonia 45
crawling 27, 69-70, 80
cryosurgery 68
CT scan 1, 29, 64, 150
cure 36, 37, 49, 111, 112, 140, 145, 156-157

D

decongestant 55
degenerative disorder
    Fahr's disease 43
    Huntington's disease 43
    Leigh's disease 43
    Wilson's disease 43
depression 76, 78

reserpine 55
retrocollis 45
risks 66
running 55, 58
Rush Institute 71

S

Scott, Dr. Alan 18, 113-114, 130
Scripps Hospital 65
secondary dystonia 30, 43
Segawa's disease 46, 140
segmental dystonia 43
selective resection and denervation 66
self-esteem 83
self-pity 73
sensory tricks 111
shaking 11, 155
Shantz, Dr. Edward 113
shoulder 9, 20, 36, 108
shout 124
side-effects 56, 60, 112, 117-118, 125
Sinemet 58, 153
sing 124
sleeping 75, 90
spasmodic dysphonia 17, 24, 45, 91, 124-126,
129, 144
abductor variety 124-126, 129
adductor variety 124, 129
spasmodic torticollis 10, 32, 37, 45
see also cervical dystonia
spasms 1, 3, 9-10, 14, 17, 47, 51, 56-57, 67,
89-90, 98, 111
spasticity 55, 129
speech 17, 19, 24, 45, 51, 68, 73, 124
spinal column 64
spinal tap 58
spirituality 87
splenius capitis 119-120

About the Author

Eugene Smith and his wife, Marcia, are long-standing volunteers for dystonia, having provided continuous services since 1987 to the Washington State Chapter of the Dystonia Medical Research Foundation. He has also written the Foundation's guide to fund-raising, *Dollars for Dystonia*, and articles for *Dystonia Dialogue*, the newsletter of the Foundation.

Before retiring in 1989 as Associate Professor Emeritus of English, University of Washington, he taught courses in writing, literature, grammar, and linguistics. He has also taught in the public schools of Oregon and Washington and has held leadership roles in the National and Washington Councils of Teachers of English and the Puget Sound Writing Program.

He is co-author of *Creating Good Landscape Design: A Guide for Non-Professionals* (1995).

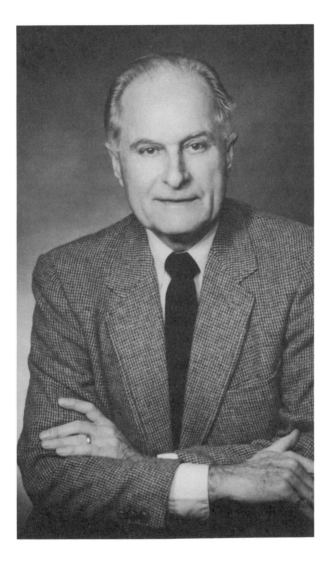

Order Form

I would like to order _____ additional copies of

Dystonia: The Disease that Distorts

Price & payment information:

US: $15.00 + $3.00 for postage & handling
CAN: $19.21 + $4.00 for postage & handling
UK: £ 9.19 + £ 3.00 for postage & handling

Amount enclosed: $_____ (US)

❏ check enclosed (please make payable to the
        Dystonia Medical Reserach Foundation)
❏ Visa ❏ MasterCard   expiration date: _____

Card number: _____

Signature: _____

Please return this form to:

Dystonia Medical Research Foundation
One East Wacker Drive, Suite 2430
Chicago IL 60601-1905
Telephone: 312-7545-0198 or 800-377-DYST
Fax: 312-803-0138   e-mail: dystfndt.aol.com